# An Introduction to Herbalism

## Herbal Remedies and Recipes for All-Natural Living

# Willa Daniels

**The Natural Path**
**An Introduction to Herbalism**
**Copyright © 2023 by Willa Daniels**



First Edition: April 2023
This edition was first published in 2023.

Cover design: Serenity Endeavors Press
Proofreader: Moniga Bogza, Trusted Accomplice

ISBN: 978-1-7377499-7-4 (Paperback)
ISBN: 978-1-7377499-6-7 (eBook)

Printed in the United States of America
Published by: Serenity Endeavors Press
**https://www.jenflanaganbooks.com/**

## *Table of Contents:*

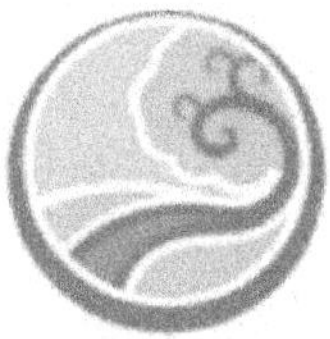

To all the herbalists out there and those trying to live a little closer to the Earth. My hat goes off to you.

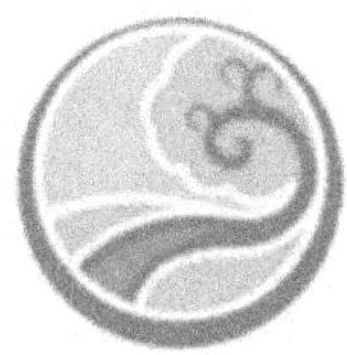

# Overview

All the recipes in this book can be made in your own home, with natural, biodegradable, and non-toxic ingredients. Most ingredients you will be able to find at your local health-food store. Mine has a nice bulk-herb section, too.

However, if you don't have one nearby, you can easily find them online. I use Amazon for a lot of my ingredients, as I can get them in bulk.

I will provide easy, step-by-step instructions with pictures wherever necessary. Sometimes, I'll add optional ways to take a recipe to the next level. Feel free to scoff at them. Only take it as far as you want to go.

All my recipes have been used by myself and others for years with no known issues outside those I make a note of. However, always test new products with caution for allergies.

These recipes are only meant to get you started and to understand the processes. Please do your own research on herbal qualities, safety, and contraindications to other medications or other herbs.

Congratulations on starting down the natural path!

*Note:* I use a few abbreviations. "Tbl" stands for tablespoon. "tsp" stands for teaspoon.

*Disclaimer:* I list a few brands I use in this booklet. I am not being paid to promote any brands. I only note them as ones I have tested and loved up to this point. Please use them only as suggestions in your own search for ingredients.

## What Brings You Here?

You may want to remove toxins and chemicals from your life. Maybe you want to save some money or try homesteading. You may be a craftsperson and want to create something fun for your family or *with* your family. To all the above, I say great. Welcome!

Occasionally, I may give options for cheaper solutions that aren't as natural but don't contain any known toxins. Alternatively, I may provide options for healthier solutions, to take it a step further and reduce chemicals. Do what works for you.

## Customization

I will give suggestions of herbs or essential oils to add to recipes for various purposes. Sometimes, they are antibacterial or anti-inflammatory. I will also give you the mix I personally use; however, some of these herbs may be harder to find or add cost. Feel free to sub it out for an herb/oil you prefer or can more easily or cheaply find.

# Reducing chemicals

It's very important to me to have a low chemical exposure. Skin is our largest organ and protects our body. I want to nourish it and my body with natural products that support its elasticity, tone, and health.

I also want to reduce the amount of chemicals used in the community, those added to the water system and runoffs. Crafting your own products also reduces the amount of waste (empty containers) in the world. Every little bit helps.

Read your labels. Just because you identify and can pronounce an ingredient, it doesn't mean it's good for you. A lot of skin care products contain petroleum and mineral oil byproducts.

Petroleum creates an illusion of moisturized skin because it repels water. But in reality, it's just not water-soluble. It seals and clogs your pores, keeping air and moisture out. If it gets into the lungs, it can cause lipoid pneumonia.

Petroleum is used as fuel for heating and electricity generation, asphalt and road oil, plastic, and other synthetic materials. It's a derivative of oil refining found coating the bottom of oil rigs, a byproduct of the oil industry.

Supposedly, the carcinogenic properties are removed in the refining processes, but as petroleum jelly can be found in a variety of different grades of purity, it's hard to say how toxic any petroleum-based product is. I personally choose not to use it on my skin.

# Herbs

For the purpose of this booklet, I'm going to refer to anything used to support the system as an herb. I realize spices and fruits, such as berries or oranges, aren't herbs, but when they're used to support your immune system, they can qualify.

Unless otherwise stated, I mean dried herbs or roots. Fresh herbs can be used in water extractions, but you need to double the amount. Fresh herbs contain water that has to be accounted for.

If your local health-food store doesn't have a bulk herb section, you shouldn't have a problem finding them online. I get several of mine from Amazon when I can't find it locally.

Try harvesting your own, either by growing it or foraging for it locally. Make sure you can clearly identify the herb. You can use a book like *Peterson Field Guide to Medicinal Plants and Herbs*. Look for a guide that has plants specific to your region. Avoid harvesting from areas that are sprayed or near road runoffs or waterways. Ensure you know local laws for foraging. Practice sustainable harvesting, only ever taking what you need or a portion of the herb patch, so it can regrow and replenish.

Herbs are cheaper when purchased by the pound, but even I am hesitant to buy that much until I've tried it first. I often buy 4oz, then move up if it's something I'm going to use often.

Starwest Botanicals, Frontier Co-op, FGO (From Great Origins), and Feel Good Organics are a few companies I buy from frequently. They offer good quality at decent prices. This doesn't mean others are not trustworthy. I've bought herbs from several different companies. These are just ones I trust consistently.

The fresher the dried herb, the more potent. Grinding the herb speeds up the aging process. Grinding isn't always necessary, depending on the use, but if you do grind, only grind right before use or packaging into teabags.

The quality and effectiveness of your products will depend on the freshness and quality of your herbs. Store them fully dried, in airtight containers, away from sunlight.

Herbal teas are great for supporting your system, but a lot of prepackaged teas have been ground and sitting on the shelf for months or years. I would still encourage people to try these before synthetic medicine, but fresher is better.

When I buy premade tea bags, I typically stick to Yogi, Stash, and Traditional Medicinals. They are organic and of fairly good quality. However, I tend to do this to try out the herb mix. Once I find a good combination of herbs, I try to recreate it with fresher dried herbs that I mix myself.

## Containers

Try using glass containers whenever possible. This is especially important for caustic ingredients like alcohol or vinegar. However, if you do choose a plastic container, try to use BPA-free ones.

Whenever possible, recycle a container. I keep three old boxes (from past Amazon orders, let's be real) on my garage shelves. When I use a good container, I clean it out and sort it for quick use.

I have purchased containers from Amazon in the past, and they work great, too. Like I said before, use what works for you. If it makes a difference to buy a cute container with a fun label, do it! I am all for a fun label.

Really, labeling is one of the best parts of making products! I get fun stickers and colored markers. I like to make up fun names for my products. My favorite one is my healing salve. I call it Tree Sap, 'cause it's green and it's fun.

I may have named my Multi-Purpose Cleaner "Molly Maid," but I'll never admit it.

*Fun tip:* Kids are more likely to use products (and get involved in making them) if they have a hand in their own mixes, labels, and names. Win!

# The Challenge

I realize it's easier to pick these products up at the local big-box store. You will likely spend more money, but you will definitely save time. Don't let the amount of time and energy discourage you, but you have to make it work for you in your life. There are stages in life when you have more time to do things like this than others. Be kind to yourself.

I challenge you to pick a recipe to start with. Read through it first, so you can get the ingredients you need and understand the process. Tackle the products you want to replace in your house one at a time.

Unless you're ready to jump headfirst, just try one recipe a month. Feel free to scale it down on your first attempt to make sure you like it.

Remember, it's about progress, not perfection. Any step you take away from chemicals and toxins is a win. Take it.

# Disclaimer

Herbs are not meant to replace medical care; they are to enhance health and support a healthy lifestyle to reduce disease.

These recipes should not substitute medical advice. Remember to do your own research and consult a trained health professional. Everybody is different, and every body is different.

Natural does not equal safe for everyone. Never treat yourself without doctor supervision. When in doubt, check with your doctor.

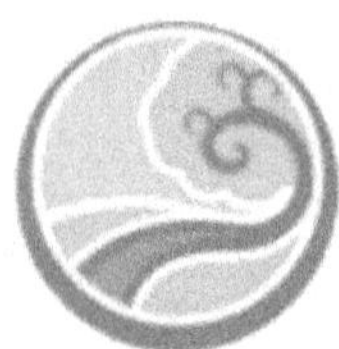

# Ingredients

Next are some highlights of the herbs used in this book. Not all are included, just a handful of my favorites with additional information about herbal health.

## Menthol

Menthol is an organic compound made from mint oils like peppermint, spearmint, or corn mint. It's a waxy, crystalline compound, which comes in either white or yellow and is solid at room temperature. A topical analgesic, this counterirritant works by causing the skin to feel cool, then warm.

*Don't:* Use on open sores. Apply more than 3-4 times daily. Use on kids younger than two, near eyes, nose, mouth, or genitals.

Wash hands well after applying.

## Vegetable Glycerin

Vegetable glycerin is a sugar alcohol made by heating triglyceride-rich vegetable fats (soybean, coconut, palm) under pressure or with a strong alkali, such as lye. The glycerin splits away from the fatty acids and bonds with the water, forming a sweet, odorless, colorless, syrup-like liquid.

It's used in food, cosmetics, and by pharmaceutical industries and may have some health benefits, like hydrating the skin or strengthening the gut.

It's added to foods to help oil- and water-based ingredients mix or to add moisture to the final product. It's also commonly used to prevent ice crystals from forming on frozen foods such as frozen yogurt and ice cream.

Glycerin is also found in toothpaste to prevent it from drying out or in soaps, lotions, and cosmetics to help keep the mixture together and add moisture.

It's generally considered safe and is naturally made. I would recommend getting a brand without soybean, as most soybeans in the U.S. are genetically modified.

I typically buy the NOW brand, which is naturally derived only from non-GMO palm, grape-seed, or coconut oils.

# Broadleaf Plantain

Plantain is used for insect and snake bites and as a remedy for rashes and cuts. It helps with itching and pain, is antibacterial, anti-inflammatory, and antitoxic. It has been medicinally used by Native Americans in poultice form to relieve the pain of bee stings, insect bites, poison ivy itch, allergic rashes, and promote healing in sores and bruises.

Plantain tea can also be used as a mouthwash to prevent sores and as an expectorant. Ongoing studies are looking into its effects on lowering blood sugar.

# Comfrey

Comfrey is also known as knitbone. It has long been used as a poultice to promote the knitting together of tissues and for cell growth. It reduces inflammation in sprains, broken bones, pulled muscles, ligaments, fractures, and osteoarthritis because it contains allantoin, which helps new skin cells grow.

# Calendula

Calendula is used for all sorts of skin issues, from dermatitis to skin abrasions. It's an excellent skin healer, reducing pain and swelling in wounds, diaper rash, burns, chapped lips, pinkeye, face redness, sore throat, and stomach ulcers.

# Garlic

This baby is my go-to when I'm feeling sick. I add fresh garlic to my food or mix some up with fresh honey and cinnamon to eat it raw.

Its ability to boost your immune system and alleviate cold symptoms is thanks to its antibacterial and antiviral properties. It's also used to reduce cholesterol and blood pressure, due to allicin, an antioxidant. Garlic has vitamins C and B6, manganese, and selenium.

# Ginger

I grab ginger at the first sign of bloating. If I've eaten something I shouldn't have (think too many fries or sweets), it calms my stomach and reduces inflammation.

Commonly used for nausea, cramps, osteoarthritis, diabetes, migraine headaches, colds, and arthritis (increases circulation).

It's loaded with antioxidants, preventing stress and damage to your body's DNA, and even increases serotonin and dopamine levels.

# Lavender

One of my favorite herbs and used widely by herbalists due to its deodorizing, antioxidant, and disinfecting qualities.

Lavender is also used to heal cuts and burns, improve sleep, support brain function, relieve pain, eliminate nervous tension, enhance blood circulation, and treat respiratory problems.

The Latin name is *lavare*, meaning "to wash."

I personally feel it's calming and relaxing, and I especially love its deodorizing qualities (think running shoes and pet beds).

Also, it's one of the few essential oils that can be used "neat," which means without dilution, without causing irritation.

# Citrus

There are so many citrus oils to use. I regularly use orange, grapefruit, and lemon; however, bergamot and mandarin are great too. Use whatever you have or whatever you like.

Citrus is used as an antibacterial, antifungal, anti-inflammatory, antidepressant (lifts your spirits), antispasmodic, antiseptic, aphrodisiac (gets the juices moving), carminative (gas reliever), diuretic (helps reduce water weight).

I regularly use citrus in my cleaning products, so you'll see them front and center in these recipes. However, as always, use what you like or what you have. I'll let you know when they're required in a recipe.

## Mint

Antimicrobial, mint is often used to freshen bad breath. Its anti-nausea qualities mean it's used for soothing the digestive tissues and gastric lining. It's used to treat IBS, bloating, and indigestion. Cooling and calming, it improves mental focus and clears respiratory tracts, which can reduce headaches and boost energy.

It's also used as an insect repellent, anti-itch, for sunburn relief, and as a fever reducer (cooling and calming, remember?).

## Rosemary

Used as a respiratory aid, antiseptic, and antimicrobial, rosemary is a good choice for bad breath, eczema, dermatitis (dandruff and dry scalp), and acne. It stimulates brain activity (energizing), so it helps with depression, mental fatigue, forgetfulness, headaches (especially associated with muscle and respiratory pain), and is used as a stress and pain reliever.

It also aids digestion, for cramps, constipation, bloating, and boosts your immune system, improves urinary tract health, and stimulates hair growth.

# Seaweeds and Algae

You know the saying "saltwater cures all wounds"? That's because practically everything from the sea has healing abilities.

From sea salt throat rinses to seaweed for antiaging serums, vitamins, and supportive nutrients, there's a world of mystery and health to be found in those salty waves.

Bladder wrack, a seaweed, although bitter, is restorative, invigorating, and known for its ability to support healthy thyroid activity. It was heavily harvested in Italy and traded through Europe for this purpose.

Wakame, another seaweed, is known for reducing cholesterol and blood pressure and increasing energy.

Sea algae, like sea lettuce, are also known for thyroid and bone health.

Sea asparagus, a succulent, is known for its vitamins A, C, and B complex, calcium, iodine, iron, and folic acid. Try it raw or cooked. I have a friend who pickles them for me, my absolute favorite way to enjoy them.

*Note:* Although all seaweed is edible, blue-green algae found in freshwater lakes is poisonous. Avoid seaweed from industrial areas as it can contain heavy metals, and inspect shoreline seaweed as it could be rotting.

# Sage

Antifungal, antimicrobial, antioxidant, antiseptic, anti-inflammatory, antispasmodic, antibacterial. This herb has it all, and it grows naturally by the sea, loving dry and sandy soils!

It's used as a cholagogue and choleretic (promotes the flow of bile), cicatrizant (anti-mark or -spot cream), depurative (discharges toxins through sweating), digestive, disinfectant, emmenagogue (regulates hormones), expectorant, febrifuge (fights infections), laxative, for the healing of old wounds (scars), and is one of the strongest stimulants (for the brain, nervous system, liver, spleen, circulatory system, and excretory system), thereby activating and optimizing functions.

Phew, that's a lot! Herbs are amazing. Thank you, Mother Nature!

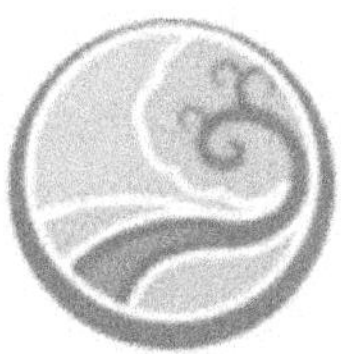

# Herb Introduction

There are several ways to reap the benefits of herbs. The simplest way is to eat them. We all know the vast number of vitamins present in foods like kale, blueberries, turmeric, and garlic. Adding beneficial herbs to your diet by sprinkling them on foods, mixing them into a smoothie, or incorporating them into a dish allows you to boost your health naturally.

Unfortunately, our foods are often modified and fertilized to the point where they don't have as many vitamins and minerals as they did years ago. It's for this reason that growing your own or buying from local farmers can improve your diet.

Your food is your fuel, but also your medicine. Nutritional medicines are how our ancestors easily maintained the balance our current generation is continuously searching for. Eat as close to the ground as possible, meaning as close to the freshly harvested source as you can with your daily life. Remember, any steps in this direction are an improvement.

Try eating some sautéed spinach or, better yet, stinging nettle! This baby is packed with protein, amino acids, vitamin K, iron, calcium, magnesium, potassium, and zinc. Just remember to wear thick gloves if you're harvesting locally. Don't eat this baby fresh and raw, either! Dry it, sauté it, or toss it in some soup. Cover with boiling water to clean it and soften its stingers, then squeeze out the liquid if sautéing. Yum!

Some herbs can even be taken in capsule form. I personally don't do this often, as infusions capture constituents from the plant that would otherwise pass through the body. Extracting them into an easily absorbed medium allows for easier access to their herbal properties.

Besides, they tend to be less fresh, ground and packaged at an unknown date. Encapsulating them yourself is an option, but time consuming. I've used capsules in a pinch, for travel or to encourage someone to try an herb, but longer term, I tend to use other methods.

I also think there's something to touching or smelling the herb I'm taking. The capsule makes it very impersonal. Part of the benefits of the mint family is captured through the olfactory sense. You remove this when you take a pill.

Dried herbs are best as they're easier to store. However, fresh is fine; just double the amount of cut-up fresh herb, as they compress substantially when dried.

Maintain whole (uncrushed) dried herbs for as long as possible, as it extends the life of the constituents in the herb.

I use a folk method for measuring my herbs. It's not precise, but plants are natural. There is a wide variation of the strength of the constituents in any given plant based on the place it's grown, the soil, the rain, and the water it gets in a season. So, for each new cutting or batch, I start with a small amount, then increase until I get the intended effect.

I give the recommended use for a 150-pound adult. Children are typically measured at a third of the adult weight and therefore would use a third of the recommended use. I use the same calculation for pets, based on their weight.

*Note:* Always do your research on herbs. Practice safety with herbs and children, pets, or pregnant/nursing mothers. Test in smaller amounts for any allergies. Herbs are not meant to replace medical care; they are meant to support and strengthen the body and to prevent disease.

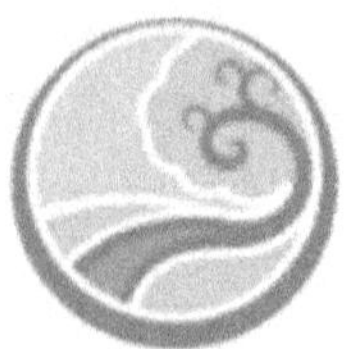

# Water Infusions

A water infusion is used to steep delicate parts of a plant, such as flowers, stems, and leaves. Another word for this is tea or tisane.

Water extracts only water-soluble constituents, like vitamins, antioxidants, sugars, polysaccharides, starches, and minerals.

Hot Water Infusion

- 1 tsp – 1 Tbl* dried herb with 8 oz very hot water.
- While water is heating, crush herbs in your hand or with a mortar and pestle to help weaken the cell walls.
- Use a steeping cup, natural teabags, or simply toss into a mason jar and strain after infusion.
- Cover to prevent loss of volatile properties.
- Steep 10-15 minutes to pull out all the valuable constituents.
- Strain the herbs out, squeezing as much liquid as possible. I use either a fine mesh sieve or cheesecloth. Compost the used herb if possible.

Cold Water Infusion

Cold water infusions are useful for mucilaginous herbs like marshmallow root, but lemon balm, peppermint, and hibiscus are nice, too.

- 1 tsp – 1 Tbl* dried herb with 8 oz cold water.

- Crush herbs to weaken the cell walls.
- Infuse for several hours to overnight in the fridge.
- Strain herbs out, squeezing as much liquid as possible. I use either a fine mesh sieve or cheesecloth. Compost the used herb if possible.

*1 tsp for tea is generally used only for enjoyment. I use about 1 Tbl when employing an herb for health benefits. Adjust down for a new batch of herbs or when testing a new herb.

*Note:* Infusions are meant to be taken every 4 hours or 3 times a day while symptoms persist. Refrigerate any unused steeped tea, covered, for up to three days.

*Concentrated infusions:* You can double or quadruple the amount of herb you use in the 8 oz of water. When concentrating, take half or a quarter of the infusion, depending on how concentrated you make it. This is helpful with bitter herbs or when taking herbs for several days in a row.

*Example:* ¼ cup of dried herb to 1 cup of water. Since this is 4 times the concentration of herb, you use ¼ cup instead of the full-cup infusion. Take every 4 hours or 3 times a day.

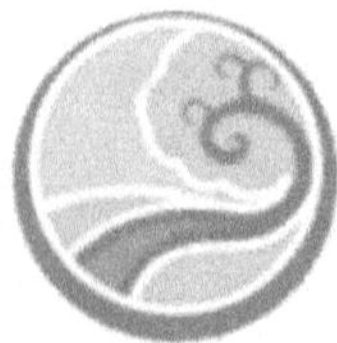

# Oil Infusions

Any oil can be infused with herbs; however, consider the oil's room-temperature state and benefits. Coconut oil is solid under 76 degrees, so mixing it with other oils may be necessary, depending on its use. Lighter oils may be desirable for massage oil.

More herbs can be used for topical use, depending on their properties. Italian herbs, like oregano and basil, are safe to use at higher ratios.

Some people double (or triple) infuse oils for an intense infusion. I've done this with dried lavender to create a lovely calming massage oil.

I generally use as much herb as I can while still allowing the oil to be stirred or shaken.

Dried herbs are the best, as fresh herbs contain water, which harbors bacteria.

- Start with 2 oz of dried herb per cup of oil.

Low-Heat Oil Infusion
- Heat the oven to 200 degrees Fahrenheit.
- Crush dried herbs to weaken cell walls.
- Add to oil in a jar or oven-safe bowl.

- Turn oven off, place oil and herb in the oven, and leave for 4-6 hours or overnight.
- Strain herbs with a fine mesh strainer or a cheesecloth, squeezing out as much oil as possible. Compost the used herb.
- Repeat if desired.

<u>Countertop Oil Infusion</u>
- Crush dried herbs to weaken cell walls.
- Place in a mason jar or other jar with a lid.
- Ensure the herbs are covered with at least an inch of oil to allow for shaking.
- Place a square of parchment paper or waxed paper over the opening, to prevent any leaching from the metal lid.
- Keep out of direct sunlight and turn to shake daily for 4-6 weeks for maximum infusion.
- Strain herbs with a mesh strainer or a cheesecloth, squeezing out as much oil as possible. Compost the used herb.
- Repeat if desired.

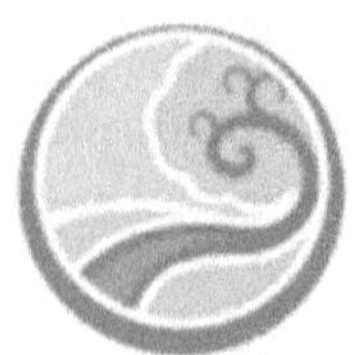

# Decoctions

Tough roots and hardy barks require more than 10-15 minutes of steeping time. Slowly simmer these to extract constituents.

A few exceptions exist, such as valerian, marshmallow, and goldenseal roots. These roots have delicate oils that can be damaged in a decoction. They are visibly smaller and thinner, hinting at a gentler steeping method.

- 1 tsp – 1 Tbl* dried herb with 8 oz water. Crush herbs to weaken the cell walls.
- Bring water and roots/bark to a boil in a <u>covered</u> pot, then lower the heat.
- Simmer for 20-45 minutes.
- Remove from the heat and strain into a heat-resistant container.

*Option*: Soak the herbs for 4 hours or overnight prior to decoction to soften the material.

- Roots and barks can be reused several times in a row if kept refrigerated, but they need to be used within a day or two. Compost the used herb.
- Larger batches can be made and stored in the refrigerator for easier processing but need to be used within a day or two as well. There are no artificial preservatives here!

*Concentrated decoctions:* You can double or quadruple the amount of herb you use in the 8 oz of water. When concentrating, you take half or a quarter of the decoction. This is helpful with bitter herbs or when taking herbs for several days in a row.

*Example:* ¼ cup of dried herb to 1 cup of water. Since this is 4 times the concentration of herb, use ¼ cup instead of the full-cup decoction. Take every 4 hours or 3 times a day.

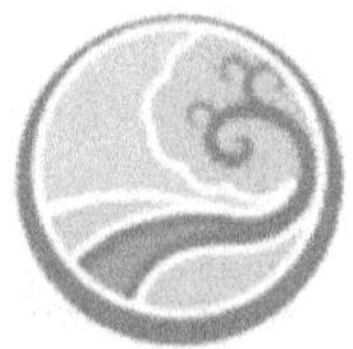

# Tinctures

Tinctures are any liquid extraction of herbal material. This is typically done with water, alcohol, glycerin, or vinegar.

Where water only extracts water-soluble constituents, alcohol extracts alkaloids, sugars, enzymes, essential oils, some minerals and vitamins, and many other plant chemicals, but it does kill mucilage, the thick, viscous coating from plants like marshmallow root, which are great for sore throats.

Glycerin and vinegar can be added to water infusions to extract additional constituents or as a preservative for those hesitant with alcohol, even though the final alcohol content is extremely low.

The typical adult usage of 1 ½ tsp = 7.4 grams (concentrated tincture), of which only 40% is alcohol, results in less than 3 grams of alcohol. To maintain its shelf-stable quality but to get rid of the alcohol, an option would be to heat the tincture in a mug just to the boiling point to burn off the alcohol. You can also add water and honey to make it easier to take.

Glycerin tinctures are called glycerites. These are used with delicate herbs, like flowers and leaves, but they don't extract as many properties as alcohol.

The same herb can produce different extractions, with different properties, based on the extraction method. Do your research or consult a professional.

I typically make alcohol tinctures with vodka, as it's a cheaper alcohol that doesn't add a lot of flavor to the tincture.

However, you can use any alcohol you like for its flavor or cost. I stick to 40% alcohol/80 proof, as it's already the perfect 40% alcohol/60% water blend, which will result in a shelf-stable tincture. If you're using a higher-proof alcohol, like moonshine, you'll want to add distilled water to the mix.

*Higher-proof alcohol:* Weighing the two and doing a little math isn't too difficult. For example, if using 45% alcohol, 100 mL of menstruum (extraction fluid) would have 45 mL of alcohol and 55 mL of distilled water. If this is too confusing, stick with the 40% alcohol.

I also use dried herbs when making alcohol tinctures, to keep the alcohol/water percentages accurate. Fresh herbs contain water that you'd have to account for to keep your tincture shelf-stable.

The benefit of using alcohol is that it's shelf-stable for 2-3 years. Glycerites and vinegar extractions are good for about 12-24 months, but glycerites require refrigeration to last as long as possible. Alcohol extractions have the longest shelf life and are relatively low in alcohol per dose, making it a good option in my book.

**Folk method (alcohol or vinegar extraction):**
- Chop or grind herbs into small pieces to expose the most surface area. The more finely ground, the more concentrated the final product.
- Fill selected jar ¾ full.

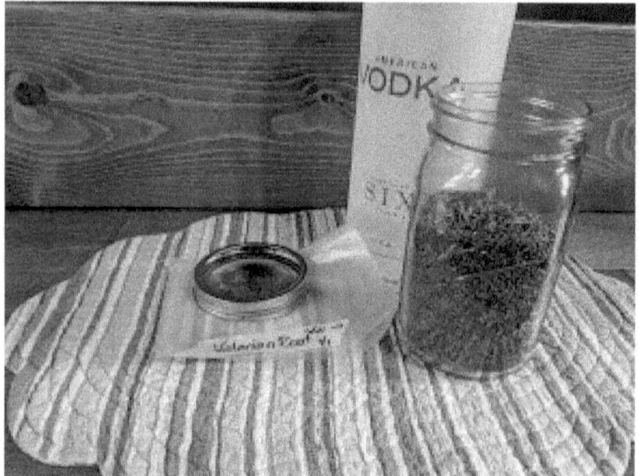

- Add vodka (or any other 40% alcohol, or vinegar) to cover the herbs completely with an inch or so of head space so you can shake it easily. Some herbs are very absorptive and require additional menstruum to be added later.

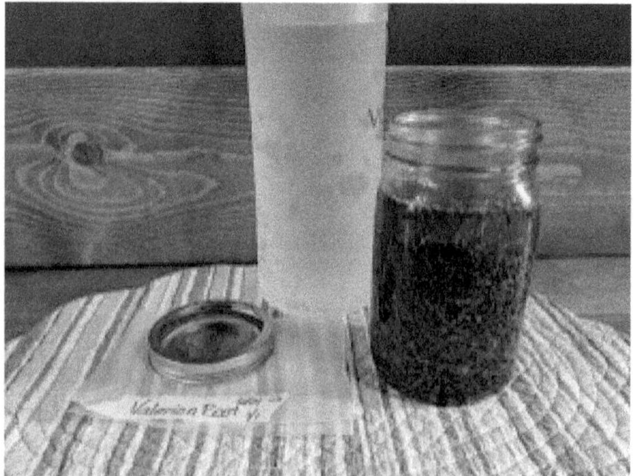

- Layer waxed or parchment paper under the lid to prevent the leaching of chemicals from the lid. Label and date.
- Store in a cool spot out of direct sunlight.
- Shake gently daily.
- Steep for 4-6 weeks.

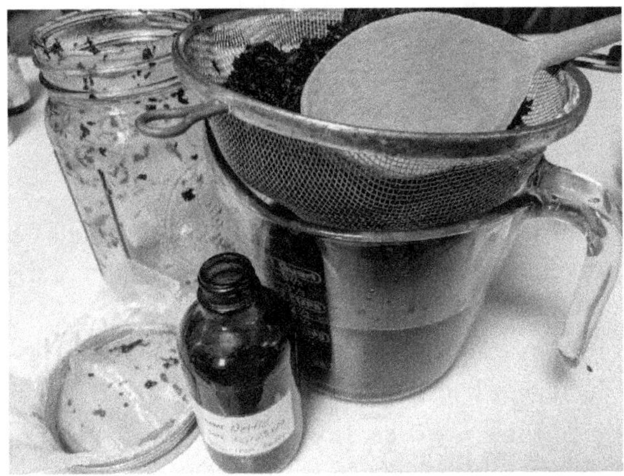

- Strain through a cheesecloth or fine mesh sieve.
- If using very finely ground herbs, you may need to use a coffee filter for the final filtering.
- Squeeze out the plant material (marc) and compost it.
- Store, labeled, in dark bottles or out of direct light.

*Note:* Alcohol and vinegar tinctures are shelf-stable for 2-3 years.

*Use:* 1 ½ tsp for an adult (concentrated, finely ground herbs) 3x daily. Adjust up as needed due to plant variability.

If you're not finely grinding your herbs, you can use closer to 3 tsp for an adult.

Remember to do your research and consult a trained health professional for specific use.

**Folk method (glycerin extraction):**
- Best for use with flowers or plant leaves.
- Fill selected jar ½ full (⅔ full if fresh herbs).

- Mix 3 parts non-GMO glycerin with 1 part water. As long as the glycerin is more than 50% of the liquid, it should preserve well. ¾ is 75%, but many people use 60% with good results.
- Pour over the plants, filling to an inch from the top.
- Layer waxed or parchment paper under the lid to prevent leaching of chemicals from the lid. Label and date.
- Store in a cool spot out of direct sunlight.
- Shake gently daily.
- Steep for 4-6 weeks. Longer time equals higher potency.
- Strain through a cheesecloth or fine mesh sieve.
- Squeeze out the plant material and compost it.
- Store, labeled, in dark bottles or out of direct light.

*Note:* Glycerites should be refrigerated for a longer lifespan and will preserve for 12-24 months.

*Use:* ¼ to ½ tsp for an adult (concentrated), 3x daily. Adjust up as needed due to plant variability.

If you're not finely grinding your herbs, you can use closer to 2-3 tsp for an adult.

Remember to do your research and consult a trained health professional for specific use.

# Valerian Root Tincture – Anxiety & Stress Relief

Often referred to as "Nature's Valium," this herb has long been used as a powerful method to reduce anxiety, insomnia, and nervous tension. It's a powerful nervine and relaxant.

During World War II, it was used to treat soldiers for post-traumatic stress disorder. It's even often used to treat dogs, children, and pregnant women, nodding to the safe nature of the herb.

Because of the strength of this herb, make sure you start with a small amount and move up. Should your arms and legs get a rubbery, heavy feeling, you're using too much and should lower subsequent usage.

This herb is extremely bitter and has a strong smell. Very good growers will produce a strong berry/floral smell with an under hint of Parmesan cheese. Older or less clean herbs will smell more strongly of stinky cheese. Either way, the tincture is a bit smelly. If it didn't work so incredibly well, I wouldn't personally use it as often as I do.

I use this as a muscle relaxer for pulled muscles to help them relax enough to heal. It also helps me get some sleep. I've used it for anxiety after a particularly stressful day. This (in glycerite form) helped my anxiety-ridden dog get through fireworks. I give it to him before they start, for best results, to ward off anxiety and stress.

If using for dogs, adjust by weight the same way you would with a child. The average use is based on a 150-pound adult. Divide accordingly. Start small and increase as needed.

To make this tincture, follow your preferred extraction method with valerian root. I prefer an alcohol extraction for the best extraction of constituents for adult use, and a glycerin extraction for pets' and children's use.

# White Willow Bark Tincture – Pain Relief

White willow bark contains salicin, which is metabolized by our bodies into salicylic acid. This is the natural chemical commercially produced as acetylsalicylic acid, the primary ingredient in commercial aspirin, with generally less stomach irritation and damage.
Extracting the single chemical for commercial, synthetic use ignores the other constituents that are thought to protect the stomach. Often, herbal remedies do not have the same side effects.

It is used for pain, including headaches, muscle pain, joint pain, menstrual cramps, RA, osteoarthritis, gout, fever, common cold, and flu. It builds up in the body, so long term use is suggested for ongoing pain relief, up to 12 weeks.

Avoid if you are allergic to aspirin, have liver or kidney disease (reduces blood flow through the kidneys), or have bleeding disorders. Stop using 2 weeks before surgery. Avoid during pregnancy and while breastfeeding. Avoid in children under 2 years of age or a child under 12 with a fever, chicken pox, or infection.

To make this tincture, follow your preferred extraction method with white willow bark. I prefer an alcohol extraction method.

# Nettle Tincture – Allergy Relief

Stinging nettle contains histamines; the very same thing that causes a histamine reaction (think hives) can also reduce your histamine response. With its anti-inflammatory qualities, it can affect several key receptors and enzymes in allergic reactions if taken when the symptoms first appear.

I use this daily during the summer for seasonal allergies, often as much as 3 times a day when symptoms are the worst.

Anti-inflammatory and calming, this tincture is a natural allergy-relief remedy also used to provide relief from water retention, aid in overall bladder health, improve diarrhea, promote hair growth, increase lactation, reduce bleeding, eczema, arthritis, and joint pain.

It's even known to stabilize the endocrine system, balancing estrogen and testosterone, making it popular for polycystic ovary syndrome support.

To make this tincture, follow your preferred extraction method with nettle. I prefer an alcohol extraction method for shelf stability when traveling.

This one is safe for pets too. I also keep nettle glycerite on hand for my pups.

Avoid if you're pregnant or breastfeeding. Use caution if you have low blood pressure, as it can lower it further.

# Echinacea – Flu & Cold Fighter

Everybody probably knows about this herb's immune system-enhancing property, but it's also been used topically to heal wounds, insect stings, and snake bites. It was the original snake oil, used to treat all venomous bites, including the brown recluse and black widow, with great results.

It's a topical disinfectant and anti-inflammatory. It also hastens skin repair, so it's also been used to fight abscesses, gum disease, boils, psoriasis, sun-related skin damage, herpes, yeast infections, and hemorrhoids.

Echinacea stops cold and flu viruses from replicating when they gain access to the tissue, and inhibits the enzymes that the virus uses connect to our cells. It stimulates the body's immune system and contains constituents that attack yeast and other kinds of fungi directly. Polysaccharides in the echinacea have an immunostimulant effect, which results in the production of leukocytes (white blood cells), which fight infection.

It's used against many infections, including the flu, UTI, yeast infections, herpes, bloodstream infections, gum disease, tonsillitis, streptococcus, syphilis, typhoid, malaria, and diphtheria.

While echinacea is an immune system-boosting herb, using it daily is not necessary. It's best used at the first signs of illness and used often. Boost your system when traveling or around sick family members. Many cases of reversing necrosis from brown recluse or snake bites exist.

Avoid if pregnant or with Hashimoto's without a doctor's recommendation due to its stimulation of the Th1 system. Use every few hours at the onset of illness. It can be applied directly to bites in tea or poultice form.

I always have a tincture of echinacea on hand for the onset of a cold/flu or insect/snake bites. It's a much stronger fighter to have on hand than a simple hot-water infusion and easier to take in multiple doses throughout the day.

To make this tincture, follow your preferred extraction method with echinacea. I prefer an alcohol extraction method for shelf stability.

# Adaptogen Tincture – Stress Fighter

Adaptogenic compounds help reduce the presence and effect of stress hormones. They work to bring the hormones of your adrenal system back into balance and overcome adrenal fatigue, a common condition of chronic stress.

By enabling the body's cells to access more energy, they help them eliminate toxic byproducts of the metabolic process and allow the body to utilize oxygen more efficiently.

Adaptogenic herbs do not alter the mood, but rather help the body function optimally during times of stress. This helps regulate cortisol excretion.

Use to reduce the effects of stress during the difficult times of your life, physically or mentally. Use with other methods of self-care to reduce stress at its core.

<u>Ingredients</u>
- 1 cup dried tulsi (holy basil)
- ½ cup cut rhodiola rosea root
- ½ cup cut ashwagandha root
- 3 Tbl reishi mushroom powder
- 2 Tbl cut American ginseng root
- 2 Tbl cut eleuthero root
- 40% alcohol (I use vodka.)
- 32 oz jar

<u>Directions</u>
- Place roots in the jar, topping them with enough alcohol to cover with at least an inch above the herbs.
- Infuse for 4-6 weeks.

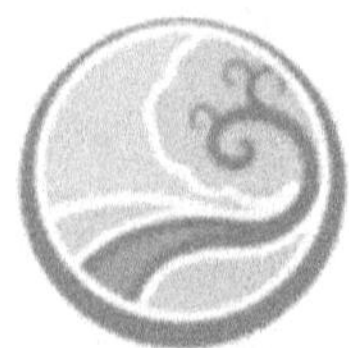

# Syrups

Syrups are very similar to glycerites in that they are sweet, easy to take, and don't break down mucilage. This makes them great for soothing herbal cough syrups.

Honey is naturally antibacterial and soothing to the throat. People used to use honey on wounds for this very purpose. It helps the wound remain moist and not attach to the dressing, but it also prevents infection.

**Folk method:**
- Best for use with flowers or plant leaves.
- Make a concentrated hot-water infusion (infusing herbs in ¼ as much water as in the hot water infusion (1 Tbl herb to 2oz of hot water), multiplying to suit your final desired amount).
- Mix 1 part of the above concentrated hot water infusion to 3 parts honey (or sugar).
- Heat gently in a double boiler, stirring gently. Avoid boiling or simmering.
- Squeeze out the plant material and compost it.
- Store, labeled, in dark bottles or out of direct light.
- Tinctures can be added to the final product if desired.

*Note:* Syrups should be refrigerated and will preserve for about a year as long as they are at least 60% honey or sugar.

*Use:* 1 Tbl for an adult every 4 hours, as needed.

# Cough Syrup

There are so many good herbs to support your respiratory system. This one uses a holy trinity (in my opinion) for upper respiratory support. However, feel free to mix your favorite cough herbs. You could try all elecampane, for example, or even all black elderberries (another popular choice). This is just a great version I've used and had good luck with.

This syrup is great to have on hand. You never know when you're going to wake up with a sore throat!

Adding the echinacea tincture at the end boosts it to support your immune system as it is known to stop diseased-cell growth in its tracks. It may still take a while to recover, but your illness won't continue to grow.

Some people prefer to use these two separately, as needed. Whip up a batch once a year, with or without the echinacea, to have ready in your refrigerator to fight respiratory problems.

Other good herbs to try would be black elderberry, hyssop, ginger, and mullein.

<u>Ingredients</u>
- 2 Tbl wild cherry bark
- 2 Tbl elecampane (helps lower respiratory)
- 2 Tbl horehound or black elderberry (helps upper respiratory)
- 4 cups filtered water
- 4 cups honey (raw and local is best)
- 5 oz echinacea tincture (optional)

<u>Directions</u>

- Decoct wild cherry bark, elecampane, and horehound in 4 cups of water. Simmer until the volume is reduced to 3 cups.
- Strain and compost herbs.
- Add 4 cups of warm (not boiling) honey, stirring gently.
- Add the echinacea tincture (made separately using the folk method), stirring gently.
- Store labeled in pourable bottles in the refrigerator.

*Option:* Substitute any of the first three herbs with 6 Tbl of your favorite cough herbs.

*Use:* ½ -1 Tbl for an adult.

# Cold & Cough Glycerite

The mix below is my favorite for cold and cough. It has more herbs than the cough syrup recipe, but it's a heavy hitter. It tonifies and strengthens your upper respiratory tract, lower respiratory tract, and immune system. The triple threat. Your upper respiratory system is your first defense to filter out offending viruses and bacteria.

Strengthening both the upper and lower systems helps prevent diseases from traveling deeper into your system. Strengthening your lung, bronchial support, and immune system promotes overall health and disease fighting.

This mix also works as an expectorant, diaphoretic, antispasmodic (improves coughs), and anticatarrhal (reduces mucus and inflammation of mucus lining). The marshmallow roots mucilage soothes sore throats.

You can make extra of this herb mix and keep it on hand for an effective cold and cough tea. Just steep a tablespoon of the mix in 8 oz of very hot water for 10-15 minutes every 4 hours. Add some raw honey to boost its healing and soothing capabilities.

<u>Ingredients</u>
- 4 Tbl marshmallow root (helps lower respiratory & soothes)
- 4 Tbl hyssop/eyebright (an expectorant)
- 4 Tbl lemon balm/lavender (a diaphoretic)
- 4 Tbl mullein/horehound (improves upper respiratory)
- 4 Tbl black elderberries/eyebright (helps sinus infections)
- 4 Tbl echinacea (boosts immune system)
- 2 Tbl thyme (helps lower respiratory)
- 2 Tbl nettle (improves allergies & is a diuretic)
- Approx. 3 cups of vegetable glycerin
- Approx. 1 cup of water

<u>Directions</u>
- Follow the glycerite extraction directions, filling a quart jar approx. ½ with crushed herbs.
- Top with a glycerin-and-water mixture, filling to an inch from the top. You will not use all the glycerin and water.
- Steep for 4-6 weeks and process as directed.

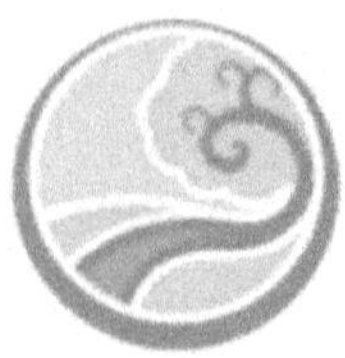

# Herbal Tonics

Tonics are used to restore health or to build the system up for general well-being. It's more of a preventative measure or to bring vigor back to the body when feeling low.

An oxymel is an herbal tonic that contains vinegar and honey and can sometimes look like a syrup, depending on how thick it's made.

## Dragon Cider

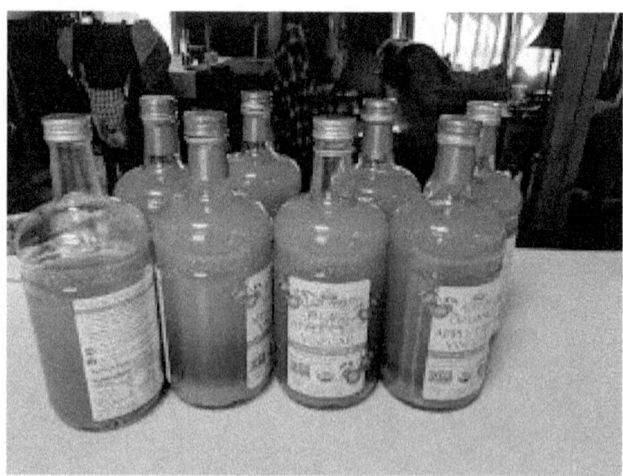

Most herbalists have a warming health tonic that will get your blood moving, like this one. Because of the controversy surrounding the copyright of the folk name, I started calling mine Dragon Cider. I think it sounds appropriate. This tonic tincture will boost your energy and immune system. Luckily, the name Fire Cider was ruled as generic and cannot be trademarked. A win for the herbalists!

Since this tonic includes honey, it could be considered an oxymel. However, I use so little that I refrain from calling it that.

We make 3 batches of this once or twice a year. Packing large jars full of ingredients and then topping them with apple cider vinegar. Then, after 6 weeks, we're straining, bottling, and setting them in our pantry for use.

Turmeric is staining, so don't wear white and try not to drip on counters or floors. We generally get it everywhere, but we get it cleaned up within an hour and haven't had any permanent stains.

I use 1 Tbl nightly after dinner, particularly when illness is going around or if I've eaten something that disagrees with me. It's good for digestion, but also keeps my immune system fully functioning. I step it up to 2 Tbl a few times a day at the first sign of a cold or flu symptom.

Vinegar is said to help regulate your acid production. If you take vinegar with food, your body is less likely to produce excess acid, causing heartburn. It seems counterproductive, but eating things like bread stimulates your body to produce more acid. If you're an overproducer, vinegar might help regulate your acid production.

<u>Ingredients</u>
- 1 cup fresh ginger (sliced or grated)

- 1 cup fresh turmeric (sliced or grated)
- 1 cup fresh horseradish (sliced or grated)
- 1 medium chopped onion
- 10 chopped garlic cloves
- 1 sliced lemon
- 1 sliced jalapeño pepper
- 2 Tbl hawthorn berries
- 2 Tbl burdock root
- 2 Tbl eleuthero
- 2 Tbl rosemary
- 3 Tbl ginkgo biloba
- 3 Tbl ginseng
- 4 Tbl honey
- 1 tsp black pepper
- Apple cider vinegar (with the mother)
- Large 64 oz jar (I use a large old pickle jar)

<u>Directions</u>
- Place all the herbs and roots in the jar, topping them with enough vinegar to cover at least an inch above the herbs.
- Infuse for 4-6 weeks.
- Play around with the ingredients. Add or subtract to make it your own. Halve the recipe to make 32 oz, or split it into two jars, or make multiple batches at once!

# Garlic Oxymel

This is a very common oxymel, used at the first sign of a cold/flu.

Garlic is an amazing antibacterial, and in a pinch, I've been known to use straight fresh minced garlic and honey. The oxymel is much easier to stomach; however, my husband thinks the fresh minced garlic and honey is delicious with a liberal sprinkling of cinnamon. The man will eat any food covered in cinnamon…or Whipped Topping.

<u>Ingredients</u>
- 1 large garlic bulb, fresh, minced
- ⅔ cup raw honey
- 1 cup apple cider vinegar
- 1 Tbl of sage, lavender, rosemary, or thyme (optional)

<u>Directions</u>
- Mix well, cap, and set in a cool, dark place for 2-3 weeks. Gently shake daily.
- Strain out the garlic if desired and store it in the refrigerator.
- Drink 2 Tbl 2-3 times a day at the onset of cold or flu symptoms.

*Note:* Do not give honey to children under 1 year of age.

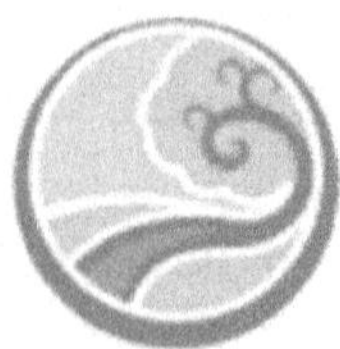

# Baths & Soaks

Baths are an easy way to use herbs topically and to support the nervous system at the same time with a healing, comforting bath.

<u>Ingredients</u>
- 2-4 oz dried herb
- 1 quart hot water (or hot bath water)
- Cheesecloth (optional)
- Ribbon or twine to tie (optional)

<u>Directions</u>
- Make a quart of very strong tea with a healing herb like calendula, plantain, or comfrey. Infuse herbs, covered, for 20 minutes.
- Strain out the herbs and add to a bath.
- Alternatively, place the herbs into a cheesecloth, tying the corners, or secure them with a ribbon or twine, and let the bath steep the herbs.
- You can even tie it to the faucet to allow the water to run through the bag, throwing it into the bath after, to further the infusion. Just make sure the water is hot enough to steep the herb and pull out the healing constituents.

<u>Herbs</u>
- Calendula, plantain, and comfrey are especially good at healing skin irritations, bruising, or strained muscles.

*Bonus:* These make charming gifts! Think about creating fun mixes for stress relief, adding pretty flowers, like rose blossoms, or colorful ribbons to the bag. Write instructions on cardstock and tie it to the bag for a personal touch.

# Bath Salts

Epsom salts aren't true salts; they are magnesium sulfate. Due to their crystalline structure, we call them salt, even without the presence of any sodium chloride. The high levels of magnesium are great for everything from relieving tension, muscle injuries, swollen joints, and body aches to headaches because magnesium can be absorbed by the skin.

You can even soak a cloth in concentrated Epsom salt water and apply it straight to strained muscles. Try a quarter cup of Epsom salts and just enough warm water to soak the cloth. Wring it out slightly and apply it, rewarming and reapplying it for 20 minutes or so. Repeat 3 to 4 times a day as needed.

Ingredients
- 4 cup Epsom salts
- 1 cup sea salt
- 1 cup baking soda
- Up to 30 drops of essential oil (optional)

Directions
- Mix everything in a large bowl or directly into a container. Stir or give the jar a good shake to mix in the essential oils.
- Store in an airtight container, like a repurposed pickle jar, in your bathroom.
- Pour approximately 1 cup into your bath.

- Soak for at least 20 minutes and let your muscles relax.

<u>Scents</u>
- Lavender & chamomile for deep relaxation.
- Citrus & eucalyptus for uplifting and invigorating baths.

*Bonus:*
- Try adding dried lavender sprigs, mint, rose petals, or citrus peels to the salts. They will infuse the salts and add to the lovely smell.
- They can be removed prior to use if you don't want the herbs in your bath.

# Milk Bath

Dead Sea salt is a sea salt from the Dead Sea used for its rich mixture of 21 minerals, such as magnesium, calcium, sulfur, bromide, iodine, sodium, zinc, and potassium. The high sulfate levels are great for detoxification and to improve circulation. The magnesium is good for its tension-relieving qualities.

<u>Ingredients</u>
- 4 cup Epsom salts or Dead Sea salts
- 4 cup powdered milk (any kind you like, but full-fat is great for moisturizing)
- 1 cup baking soda
- 6 Tbl raw honey
- 4 tsp carrier oil (I use almond or olive)
- Up to 30 drops of essential oil (optional)

<u>Directions</u>
- Mix everything in a large bowl.

- Use a whisk or your fingertips to work the honey and oils into the other ingredients. I like to use my fingertips, so I can break up the pieces into smaller beads.
- Store in an airtight container, like a repurposed pickle jar (it probably sounds like I eat a lot of pickles), in your bathroom.
- Pour approximately 1 cup into your bath.
- Soak for at least 20 minutes and feel your stress melt away!

<u>Scents</u>
- Lavender & chamomile for deep relaxation.
- Calendula for skin healing and pampering.
- Geranium & lavender are also great scent options.
- *My favorite is 20 drops calendula and 10 drops clary sage.

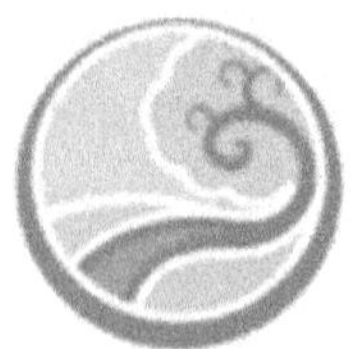

# Steams

Steams are used for upper respiratory issues, facials, and relaxation. This blend is good for all three. thyme, marjoram, and mint are good for upper respiratory issues and are antibacterial. Chamomile is relaxing and calms down inflamed tissues (sinuses or skin).

Ingredients
- 1 Tbl chamomile
- 1 Tbl thyme
- 1 Tbl marjoram
- 1 Tbl mint
- 2 quarts hot steamy water

Directions
- Use a small saucepan to bring the water to a boil.
- Transfer to a cooler bowl on a table where you can sit with your head over it.
- Add your herbs, covering the bowl while you get a towel over your head and position your face over the bowl.
- Remove the lid carefully so you don't burn yourself with the steam, but try to catch as much of the initial steam as possible as it is the most potent.

*Options:* Substitute the herbs with 4 Tbl of your choice in herbs. Peppermint and camphor have menthol in them, making a more potent sinus pressure-relieving steam. Use with caution.

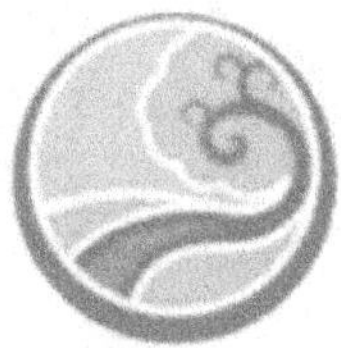

# Topical Oils, Salves & Balms

We already talked about infusing oils. The next step is to add a little beeswax to thicken the infused oil and help it stay on the skin. Beeswax is also an emollient and seals in the moisture, maintaining this barrier.

Think about the consistency of lip balm and how it maintains a layer of moisture that stays put on the lip.

The salve can be as hard or soft as you want, depending on your purpose.

You can leave the beeswax out entirely for a powerful massage oil. Lavender and chamomile are very relaxing. Citrus peels make an invigorating circulatory system-reviving rub.

Follow the directions to make an oil infusion, using your preferred method.

Warm the infused oil in a double boiler. I use a Pyrex glass measuring cup so I can easily pour the finished product into containers.

Place the Pyrex cup in a small saucepan filled with water. Heat the saucepan over the stovetop on medium so the water warms the sides of the Pyrex cup slowly.

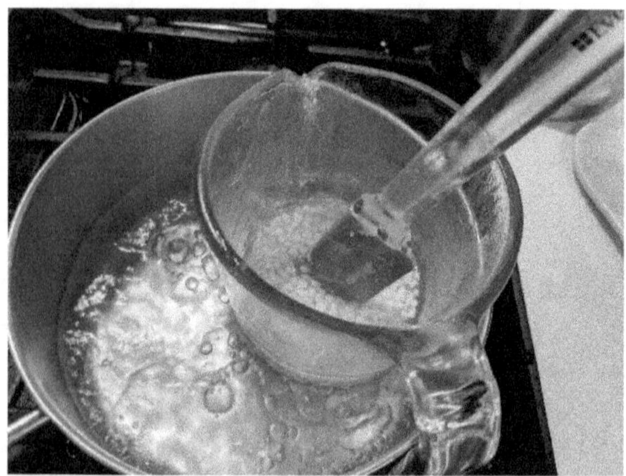

Add approximately 1 ounce of beeswax per cup of oils and stir until it melts completely. I use beeswax pastilles as they are easier to pour and work with, but you can buy beeswax in blocks and shave or chop off your desired amount.

There's no real difference between white or yellow beeswax. I prefer white as I use it to thicken my deodorant and body butters and prefer it to be colorless. However, if you like the yellow shade, use it.

To test the thickness of your salve, dip a knife into the mixture (or use your spoon) and place it in the fridge for 5-10 minutes to cool. Run your finger over the salve to test the thickness.

Add more wax to thicken it further. If it's already thicker than you hoped, add a little extra infused oil or plain carrier oil (almond or olive) to thin it out.

Cool the oil a little (10-20 minutes) before pouring it into plastic containers, but don't wait until it cools all the way, as it won't pour nicely.

Make sure you label your containers! Pick fun names.

# Healing Salve (Tree Sap)

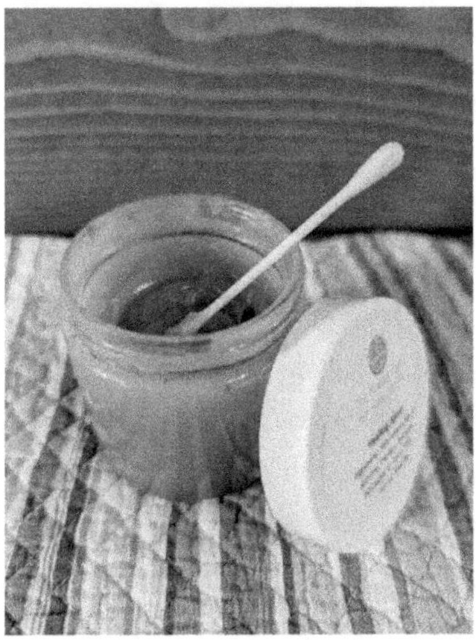

This is probably my most-often-used recipe and my favorite. I use it anytime anyone gets a cut or a scrape. I use it under bandages and to take away the sting from bug bites.

It encourages healing and has antibacterial and anti-inflammatory qualities.

I keep a quart jar of infused oil on hand so I can make more salve whenever I run out. I thicken it with beeswax and pour some into several tiny jars. The rest goes into a few larger jars kept in the bathrooms and kitchen.

The little jars are tucked into travel bags and bedrooms or in my husband's workshop. I always have extras to give to friends.

My husband gave one to his brother, who unfortunately, cut off the tip of his finger. He used this daily, and I was surprised to find no redness at all on his finger after only 2 weeks.

<u>Ingredients</u>

- 2 Tbl dried comfrey leaf (promotes growth of skin cells)
- 2 Tbl dried plantain leaf (pain reliever, antibacterial/antitoxic)
- 2 Tbl dried calendula flowers (reduces swelling and pain)
- 1 tsp dried St. John's wort
- 1 tsp dried echinacea
- 1 tsp dried yarrow flowers (stops bleeding) (optional)
- 1 tsp dried rosemary (astringent) (optional)
- 1 ½ - 2 cups olive oil (antioxidant)
- 1-pint jar
- ¼ cup beeswax pastilles

<u>Directions</u>

- Put the herbs in the jar. Top with enough olive oil to cover completely with at least an inch of head space, and shake.
- Infuse the oil with the method of your choice.
- Strain and compost the used herb.
- Warm the oil in a double boiler, adding the beeswax. Use more or less to thicken to your personal preference. Stir until it melts.
- Pour into containers and label.
- Make sure you only use clean hands or a clean applicator like a cotton swab to dip into the jar.

# Hemp Pain Reliever Rub

This recipe is a nonmenthol pain reliever for general aches and pains. It's anti-inflammatory and good for arthritis.

Hemp oil is known for its ability to improve joint pain but does tend to have a shorter shelf life. Because of this, I always use the cold-oil infusion method and infuse this in the refrigerator to extend it as long as possible.

Ingredients

- 1 cup grated ginger
- 3 Tbl frankincense resin beads or powder
- 3 Tbl green tea
- 3 Tbl ground dried peppermint
- 6 Tbl cinnamon chips
- Quart-sized mason jar
- Quart of hemp oil
- ½ cup Epsom salts (magnesium)
- 1 Tbl arnica oil
- 20 drops cinnamon essential oil (optional)
- 45 drops peppermint essential oil (optional)
- 30 drops frankincense essential oil (optional)
- 20 drops ginger essential oil (optional)
- 20 drops helichrysum essential oil (optional)

Directions

- Put the herbs in the mason jar. Top with enough hemp oil to cover completely with at least an inch of head space and shake.
- Infuse the oil with the cold-oil infusion directions for 4-6 weeks.
- Strain and compost the used herb.
- Add Epsom salts, arnica, and essential oils (if using) after straining and shake lightly.
- I store the bulk of the infused oil in the fridge to extend its life. A smaller, 2-oz bottle, of oil sits in my bathroom cabinet to rub onto sore muscles after a shower. Or use it directly from the fridge for a cooling massage oil.

# Menthol Muscle Rub

This muscle rub is great for muscle sprains and strains. It has menthol to take the oils deeper into the muscle and has a nice minty scent.

This recipe includes quite a few essential oils. After playing around with different ones, I've found these to be the most effective. Some can be a little expensive. Feel free to play around with the mix and do what's best for you.

I find it very useful for arthritis, lower back, and neck pain. This rub is a topical analgesic for deep muscle pain relief.

Make sure you wash your hands well after applying, *especially* before you rub your eyes or use the restroom!

<u>Ingredients</u>

- ½ shea butter
- ¼ cup coconut oil
- 2 Tbl olive oil
- 8.5 gr beeswax
- 1 Tbl borage seed oil (anti-inflammatory)
- 1 vitamin E capsule
- 20 drops arnica (helps with bruising, swelling)
- 1 Tbl glycerin
- 1 tsp menthol
- 20 drops birch/wintergreen essential oil (contains methyl salicylates to relieve sore and fatigued muscles, is anti-inflammatory, offers pain relief, eliminates toxins)
- 20 drops blue tansy essential oil (calming, soothing, relaxing, reduces inflammation)

- 20 drops German (blue) chamomile essential oil (reduces pain by calming and sedating nerves, antihistamine, is anti-inflammatory)
- 10 drops camphor essential oil (cooling, offers pain relief, increases blood flow)
- 10 drops peppermint essential oil (cooling, calming for sore muscles)
- 10 drops vetiver essential oil (calms imbalances)
- 10 drops Helichrysum essential oil (anti-inflammatory, free-radical scavenging, heals nerves, joints, and muscle tissue, arthritis, eliminates toxins, reduces bruises, prevents blood clots, stimulates cellular regeneration)
- 10 drops geranium essential oil (improves circulation, anti-inflammatory, soothing)
- 2 drops ylang-ylang essential oil (soothes inflammation and irritation)
- 8 oz container (or two 4oz containers)

Other good essential oils to use:
- Eucalyptus (anti-inflammatory, antispasmodic, antiseptic, analgesic, soothes nervous tension)
- Osmanthus (contains polyphenols to relieve fatigue, stress, and depression)

<u>Directions</u>
- Warm shea butter, coconut oil, olive oil, and beeswax in a double boiler. Stir until beeswax is fully melted.
- Remove from heat, stir in the borage seed oil, arnica, vitamin E, and glycerin.
- Let the mixture cool for 10 minutes before adding menthol and essential oils. Menthol is potent. It will open your sinuses!
- Stir and pour into containers.

*Note:* Menthol is often solid at room temp. Do not microwave! Place the menthol jar in a heat-resistant bowl and pour boiling water into the bowl around the jar. The hot water will gently warm it enough to pour.

# Vapor Rub

This petroleum-free salve is made from a base of coconut oil and beeswax, enriched with a blend of essential oils such as menthol, camphor, and peppermint.

It's great for reducing coughing or for sinus and respiratory pain relief due to colds or allergies. Apply liberally to the chest and throat after a warm Epsom bath. The menthol vapors will aid in opening and easing the respiratory system.

Apply it to the bottom of the feet to help pull out toxins (cover with socks). Add a teaspoon or two into a large pot of water for steam inhalation.

Ingredients
- 7 Tbl coconut oil
- 21 g beeswax
- ½ tsp menthol
- 30 drops peppermint (menthol, respiratory relief, invigorating, pain relief, expectorant, antispasmodic, decongestant)
- 30 drops camphor (menthol, decongestant, respiratory relief)
- 10 drops rosemary (throat congestion, immune system, reduces fatigue)
- 5 drops eucalyptus (improve oxygen flow)
- 5 drops lemon (respiratory function, uplifting, immune system)

- 3 drops tea tree (fights infections)
- 4 oz container

Other good oils to use:
- Laurel leaf (helps respiratory system, expectorant, decongestant, strengthens immune system)
- Cardamom (helps respiratory system)
- Ravintsara (calming, improves muscular aches and pains, boosts immune system, aids sleep)

<u>Directions</u>
- Warm coconut oil and beeswax in a double boiler. Stir until the beeswax is fully melted.
- Remove from heat, and let the mixture cool for 10 minutes before adding the menthol and essential oils. Remember, menthol is potent; it will open your sinuses (kinda the point)!
- Stir and pour into containers.

*Note:* Remember to warm the menthol (to liquefy it) in a heat-resistant bowl by pouring boiling water into the bowl around the jar.

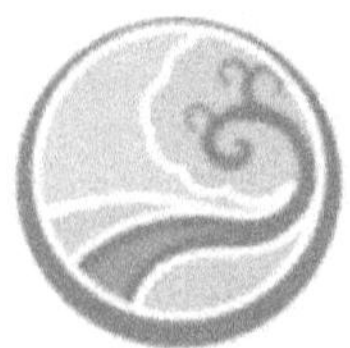

# Tea

I spent my high school and college years in the Florida Panhandle. If you'd have asked me 10 years ago, I would have told you that I didn't like tea at all. All I had been exposed to was syrupy-sweet iced tea. I personally still don't like that.

I have found that I prefer iced herbal teas, drank for pleasure. Give me some hibiscus petals with citrus peels, cold-infused, strained, and poured over ice, and I'm a happy girl. Green tea with a mashed peach or pear has a similar effect. Toss in some nettle or red clover for their benefits, and baby, you're golden.

I'm a coffee drinker, through and through. I wholeheartedly love the smell and taste of the beautiful bean and believe that *some* caffeine can actually be good for you. However, as an herbalist, I also realize that too much caffeine can cause a boatload of issues, from hormone balancing, to sleep and anxiety. I personally stick to two cups of coffee a day, three if I'm just soaking in the morning and unable to move on.

Most afternoons, I enjoy a hot herbal tea for its nutritional benefits, whether it's a stress relief from a busy day or to get some vitamins and nutrients. I typically enjoy these teas, but it's mainly because I know they're doing good things for me. I can't explain it any other way. They don't have a strong taste but are warm and comforting.

In the evening, I often enjoy herbal coffee or masala chai. Funny how, so many years later, this dislike of tea has turned into 2+ cups a day. I still look forward to my hot cup of joe when I roll out of bed in the morning, but nowadays, it's for pure enjoyment, not for energy or to prevent a headache.

These recipes are my favorite for their nutritional value. They aren't all made for their taste, but they will help when you need it. Remember, you can always make a concentrated infusion or a tincture (depending on the herbal constituents you desire) if you hate the taste but want the effect.

Holistically, I believe there is value to tea. Holding a warm cup in your hand adds a layer of mental and physical well-being that you can't get from a capsule or tincture. This is especially true for digestive tonics and cold-fighting blends. Remember, health doesn't come from a singular source. We are beings with many needs. Treat the body, mind, and spirit.

I often use a metal or silicone tea steeper; however, I buy empty unbleached paper tea bags that I can prefill for friends or traveling. I also keep some unbleached cotton tea bags on hand for the turmeric tonic and masala chai. The ground herbs in those recipes clog the paper tea bags too much to drain well. It still works, but not as easily.

A supplemental dose is 1 Tbl steeped in very hot water for 15-20 minutes.

Remember, these recipes are just to get you started. If you can't find an herb or you don't like the taste of it, leave it out. It's as easy as that. Add notes or create your own recipes based on the info in this booklet and your own research.

# Turmeric Tonic

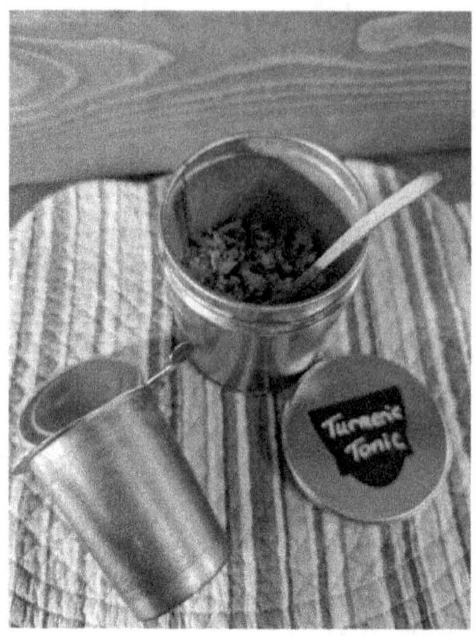

My favorite digestion tonic, this tea is also a detox with anti-inflammatory benefits. I use this if I eat something I shouldn't have and feel bloated. I also drink this to boost my immune system if I feel a cold or flu coming on.

It's lightly spicy from the ginger root and full of flavor from the turmeric. Be careful of drips or where you set your tea strainer/tea bag as turmeric stains!

Steep in very hot coconut milk for a treat. Sweeten with raw honey as desired.

- 6 Tbl powdered or dried turmeric
- 6 Tbl powdered or dried ginger root
- 4 Tbl powdered cinnamon or cinnamon chips
- 4 Tbl fennel
- 2 Tbl tulsi (holy basil)
- 2 Tbl dandelion root

- 1.5 Tbl black pepper (helps the absorption of the
  curcumin in the turmeric)

*Note:* The powdered herbs clog paper filters. Try cotton filters,
a tea steeper, or simmer on the stove and strain.

# Golden Milk

This drink tastes like a dessert, but it has all the health benefits
of the turmeric tonic; it's just a little bit more decadent and a bit
fussier, preferring fresh, toasted spices. It's still great for
detoxification, as anti-inflammatory, and good to use when
you're fighting a cold or flu.

Use fresh turmeric and ginger, if possible. Jarred is second best
and, finally, ground if that's what you have.

- 1 Tbl grated turmeric
- 1 Tbl grated or sliced ginger
- 1/2 tsp ground cinnamon
- 1/8 tsp ground black pepper
- 2 cups milk (coconut milk is preferred)
- 1 Tbl raw honey

<u>Directions</u>
- Heat herbs in a saucepan over medium heat until
  toasted and fragrant (1-3 min).
- Add milk and honey, bring to a boil, and simmer for 10
  minutes.
- Strain in a fine mesh sieve (if using fresh herbs) and top
  with a dash of cinnamon. Froth with a blender or wand
  for foamy fun.
- Store any extra covered in the refrigerator for up to 5
  days.

# Red Raspberry Leaf

This herb is a well-known uterus tonifier, which means it tones and strengthens your uterus organ. It's safe to use during pregnancy. I have given this herb to several pregnant friends to help prepare their uterus for pregnancy.

During your menstrual cycle, this tea will help balance hormones, especially if you have elevated estrogen. I find it helps with cramps, mood swings, and to normalize your cycle.

Because this herb is also an astringent, it's very helpful when fighting diarrhea, but it's also high in antioxidants, calcium, iron, magnesium, manganese, niacin, selenium, vitamins A and C.

# PMS Blend

This blend helps balance hormones, emotions, and reduce cramping during your menses.

- 4 Tbl dong quai
- 4 Tbl dandelion root
- 2 Tbl wild yam
- 2 Tbl astragalus
- 1 Tbl licorice root

<u>Other good herbs to use</u>
- Black cohosh: Used for menopausal hot flashes, night sweats, painful periods, depression, and anxiety. Use with consistency for full effect. Don't use if pregnant.
- Chasteberry: Used to normalize hormones, PMS, and for infertility. Don't use if taking dopamine-blocking meds.

For:

- Night sweats: Try red clover, dong quai, sage, and St. John's wort (also an antidepressant).
- Spotting when not in cycle: lady's mantle.
- Try adding in a stress reliever like passionflower, chamomile, or blue vervain.

# Stress Relief

Most of these herbs are nervines, meaning they help support the nervous system. Drink this tea when you're trying to fight stress or having trouble sleeping.

I added the two herbs at the bottom as optional. Valerian root is a bit stinky, and I personally don't like the taste of it. I typically use it as a tincture when needed. But it's very powerful, and some people have no issues drinking it as tea.

Blue vervain doesn't taste good, either, but it's nowhere near as strong. It's also harder to find (and good to have on hand against vampires).

Use what works for you. Play around with it.

- 4 Tbl chamomile
- 4 Tbl passionflower
- 4 Tbl oat straw
- 2 Tbl tulsi (holy basil)
- 1 Tbl lemon balm
- 2 Tbl blue vervain (optional)
- 2 Tbl valerian root (optional)

# Mood Lifter

This tea is pink, with a light lemony flavor, and happy to look at. It helps form a sunny disposition. Try this hot or iced.

- 2 Tbl lemon balm
- 2 Tbl hibiscus
- 2 Tbl rose hips

# Cold & Cough

This mix is very similar to the cold & cough syrup. The herbs are soothing and support the upper respiratory system, the lower respiratory system, work as an expectorant, and boost the immune system, making them perfect when fighting a cold.

Add a teaspoon of raw honey when steeping. Drink it 3-4 times a day while symptoms persist.

- 4 Tbl marshmallow root
- 4 Tbl hyssop
- 4 Tbl mullein
- 4 Tbl lemon balm
- 2 Tbl peppermint
- 2 Tbl echinacea
- 2 Tbl fennel
- 2 Tbl nettle
- 2 Tbl thyme
- 2 Tbl black elderberries
- 1 Tbl hawthorn berries

# Honey Chamomile

One of the few teas I drink purely for comfort. Chamomile is a great stress reliever, but in this mix, I most often drink it just for the taste. I grow my own chamomile and love the sweet, almost musty scent of the sunny flower.

- 1 cup chamomile flowers
- 2 Tbl orange peel
- 1 Tbl vanilla bean

# Fall Apple

This tea screams fall. There are some mild relaxation herbs in this mix, and cinnamon and orange are good for the immune system and the coming colder temps, but mostly, it's an enjoyable blend to remind us of the changing season.

- 3 Tbl chamomile
- 3 Tbl dried apple chips (dry your own thinly chopped slices in an oven at 200 for 2-4 hours)
- 3 Tbl cinnamon chips
- 2 Tbl hibiscus
- 1 Tbl orange peel
- ½ Tbl licorice root

# Herbal Coffee

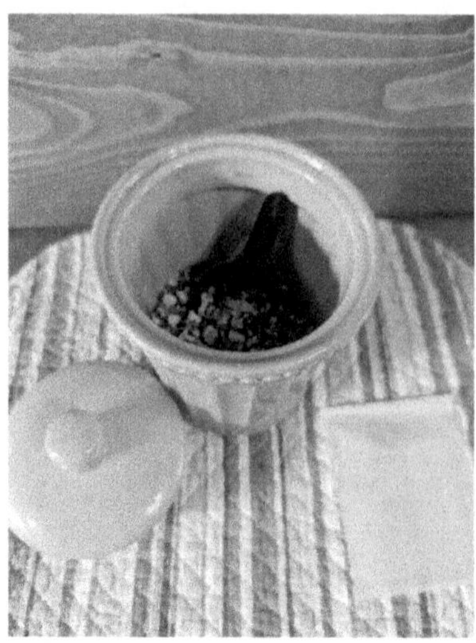

As a coffee drinker, I'll be clear that this doesn't taste like coffee. It is bitter and rich and has a taste profile similar to coffee, but it's got some great benefits as well. I don't get jittery when I drink it and would go as far as to say that I feel "nourished." It's a feeling of well-being.

Pau d'arco is used as an anticancer supplement and is antimicrobial, especially beneficial against candida. It's used for diabetes, inflammation, gastritis, liver ailments, asthma, bronchitis, joint pain, hernias, etc.

Burdock is good for the liver, and reishi mushroom is used for boosting the immune system, among other things.

- 8 Tbl pau d'arco bark
- 5 Tbl dandelion root
- 5 Tbl chicory root
- 2 Tbl burdock root
- 2 Tbl reishi mushroom powder

- 1.5 Tbl dried mushroom

# Masala Chai

This delicious, spicy tea is traditionally served warm, lightly sweetened, with coconut milk. Ginger and clove support digestion after dinner. I use all ground herbs to make this tea simple to make.

Chai means "tea" in Hindi. Masala refers to the spice blend that typically accompanies their tea leaves. It varies from region to region. This is my favorite mix.

- 1 cup loose-leaf black tea
- 4 Tbl ground cinnamon
- 4 Tbl ground ginger
- 3 Tbl ground cardamom
- 2 Tbl ground cloves
- 1 Tbl ground nutmeg

*Add a shot of espresso or a spoonful of espresso powder for Dirty Chai, my husband's favorite!

# Nettle

Nettle is used to calm allergic reactions. However, most of the time, I use it in tincture form for this purpose. This is mainly because, during the summer months, I'm taking it 1-3 times a day. I would be very tired of nettle after 2-3 months of that.

However, if I've forgotten to take it that morning or am traveling, I can easily take dry nettle with me for a quick cup of tea.

Nettle also makes a great diuretic, improves liver and kidney functions (detox), is high in chlorophyll (digestion), and contains vitamins A and C, calcium, potassium, magnesium, iron, and amino acids.

# Dandelion Root

This tea is readily available everywhere. I harvest dandelion roots in my yard in the spring, away from run-offs and pet areas. Don't harvest your own if you spray your yard with chemicals.

I enjoy this tasty root. It has a warm, nutty taste that increases drastically when you toast it. I clean and chop up the roots, then dry them in my oven at 200 degrees Fahrenheit. This also toasts the root, making it especially tasty.

Drink a cup of this tea after a night of overeating or drinking, as it is a detoxifier and liver tonifier. Your liver will thank you!

# Daily Vitamins

These herbs give you tons of vitamins, minerals, and nutrients to support a healthy life. Either cycle through these herbs in daily teas as needed or make a mix to drink daily.

- 3 Tbl alfalfa (contains vit A, K, and chlorophyll)
- 3 Tbl dandelion leaf (contains calcium, iron, vit A, enriches the blood to fight anemia, strengthens the liver, helps digestion, constipation, urinary tract)
- 3 Tbl parsley (contains vit C, folic acid)

- 2 Tbl catnip (contains vitamins A, B, and C, calcium, iron, magnesium, manganese, phosphorus, potassium, selenium, and sodium)
- 2 Tbl peppermint (contains calcium, magnesium, phosphorous, iron, niacin, potassium, riboflavin, thiamine, vit A, amino acids, helps digestion, nausea, circulation, abdominal gas, bloating, muscle spasms, is diaphoretic)
- 2 Tbl plantain (contains beta carotene, vit C, calcium, combats indigestion)
- 2 Tbl reishi Mushroom (supports the heart, immune system, improves blood pressure, cholesterol, liver, kidney, respiratory system, fights viral infections, cancer, offers chemo support, and is antiaging)
- 2 Tbl ginkgo biloba (contains calcium, iron, vit C, helps circulation, is antiaging)
- 1 Tbl nettle (detoxes, helps liver, kidney, digestion, contains chlorophyll, vit A, C, minerals, calcium, potassium, magnesium, iron, amino acids)
- 1 Tbl echinacea (strengthens the immune system, stops viral infections from multiplying, and reduces their symptoms)
- 1 Tbl sage (contains zinc, calcium, magnesium, potassium, thiamine, vit A, helps digestion, inflammation, headaches, nervous system strengthening)

*Bonus:*

*Women:*

- Red raspberry (hormone balancing, reduces estrogen dominance, migraine relief, contains antioxidants, calcium, iron, manganese, magnesium, niacin, selenium, vit A, vit C)

- Red clover (contains chromium, calcium, magnesium, niacin, potassium, phosphorous, thiamine, vit C, supports estrogen production, fights inflammation, digestion, pain, used to tonify and support female organs)
- Damiana (hormone balancing, used for menopause, and premenstrual syndrome)

*Men:*

- Saw palmetto (combats asthma, benign prostatic hypertrophy, pelvic pain syndrome, prostate cancer, stress)
- Tribulus terrestris (Gokshura) (improves muscle strength, cholesterol, hormone levels, urinary tract health, reduces blood sugar, balances testosterone)
- Damiana (helps hormone balancing, dyspepsia, diarrhea, constipation, used to tonify and support male organs)

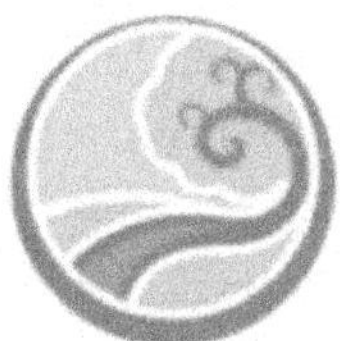

# Honey Drops

These honey drops are shelf-stable, so they're easier to use than water infusions. You can upcycle and decorate an old mint tin. The honey's sweetness encourages kids to use the herbal preparation.

The sugar in the honey acts as a natural preservative. Each serving doesn't contain a huge amount of sugar, and because it isn't a form of bleached, processed sugar, it makes it a healthier alternative in my book. Honey is healing, a natural antibacterial, and helps soothe the throat.

Ingredients

- ¾ cup raw honey
- ½ cup very concentrated water infusion or decoction of choice
- Slippery elm bark powder for dusting

Directions

- Use 4-6 Tbl dried herbs for an ultra-strong concentration due to the size of the drops.
- Strain and measure your water infusion/decoction.
- Add honey. Cook down to a hard boil, stirring constantly for 20-30 minutes. Don't let the mixture foam, or it could burn.

- Hard-crack test: Drop small pieces of the sugar mixture into a cup of ice-cold water. Once it's cold, fish it out with a fork. If it's soft to the touch or the threads are bendable, let the sugar cook longer.
- Use a silicon candy mold or drop little pools onto a coconut-oiled cookie sheet or parchment paper to harden and cool.
- Once they cool slightly, you can shape them more if desired. Oil your hands and work quickly. Be careful with the heat.
- Roll in the slippery elm bark powder after it cools, and store in a tin or other container. Slippery elm bark will keep them from sticking together, especially if they don't harden as much as desired.

*Note:* Use caution. Could be a choking hazard for small children.

# Cough Drops

I make a batch of these cough drops every few years to keep on hand. The sweetness encourages kids to use the herbal preparation. The drops are shelf-stable, so they're easy to use and last quite a while.

Honey and slippery elm bark both help soothe the throat.

<u>Ingredients</u>
- ¾ cup raw honey
- ½ cup very concentrated water infusion of:
  - 1 Tbl hyssop
  - 1 Tbl marshmallow root
  - 1 Tbl echinacea
  - 1 Tbl black elderberries

- o   1 Tbl grated fresh ginger (optional – for warming and antibacterial qualities)
  - o   ½ cup water
- Slipper elm bark powder for dusting

<u>Directions</u>
- Follow the directions for honey drops.

# Ginger Drops – Digestion

These drops are great for digestion issues, whether from gas, bloating, or indigestion. I keep them in a drawer at work and in my travel bag. We often don't eat as healthy at work or when traveling, when we don't have control over how fresh our food is or how many preservatives there are.

<u>Ingredients</u>
- ¾ cup raw honey
- ½ cup very concentrated water infusion of:
  - o   1 Tbl grated fresh ginger
  - o   1 Tbl peppermint
  - o   ½ Tbl oregano
  - o   ½ Tbl tarragon
  - o   1 tsp ground clove
  - o   ½ cup water
- Slippery elm bark powder or reishi mushroom powder for dusting

<u>Directions</u>
- Follow the directions for honey drops.

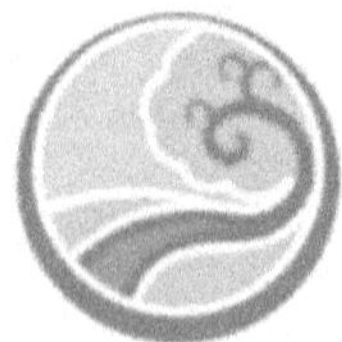

# Essential Oil Introduction

There's a lot of information out there today about essential oils. Some claim to cure everything from cancer to mental disorders. I won't make any of these claims, but they are a great way to get into plants and herbs due to the ease of use and the length of their useful life.

## What Are Essential Oils?

Essential oils are concentrated hydrophobic liquids containing volatile chemical compounds from plants. Basically, they are concentrated plant extracts that retain the natural smell and "essence" of the plant.

They are not fatty oils, as we typically know oils to be, meaning they usually evaporate completely, without residue.

Typically, they are derived by distillation. If obtained through a chemical process, they aren't considered to be true essential oils.

Fragrance oils aren't essential oils. They will be cheaper, are typically mixed with other carrier oils, and are used for soaps, candles, and cosmetics.

# Benefits of Essential Oils

Essential oils are shelf-stable, meaning they don't have to be refrigerated. However, a few, like red raspberry seed, go rancid within a year, so I refrigerate mine. Most will last 2+ years without spoilage.

They are easy to transport and use. I've been known to add a few drops of carrier oil to my hand, top it with a few drops of essential oil, and apply it to myself or my kids in a pinch for a cold or flu.

EOs are aromatic, with a compact structure, and can easily circulate in the air. They are fat-soluble, so they can enter the brain tissue to deliver their therapeutic benefits directly.

Most substances that cross the blood-brain barrier are chemicals, pollution, and toxins. EOs are one of the few good substances with this ability. This is one reason they are so widely used in aromatherapy, for detoxification, hormone production, to improve memory storage, emotional balance, and more.

If you get a headache while using one, discontinue use immediately. You could personally have a reaction to the specific essential oil, or it could be the brand.

They are especially good at penetrating the skin, nerve pathways, and cellular walls. It's no wonder they are so widely used today.

# Brands

I'm not a big proponent of brand names; however, I do trust some companies more than others. I've done a lot of research on essential oils and personally feel no one company makes the best of all essential oils.

Some companies make superb peppermint oil, but not an amazing clary sage, for example. Most companies have a niche. Pay attention to online reviews. Try them out for yourself. See what you like.

I don't always buy the most expensive brand. Occasionally, I do. Sometimes, I buy cheaper oils for soap making. Usually, I buy one with a higher amount of positive reviews and a mid-range price.

A few brands I typically trust are NOW, doTERRA, Healing Solutions, Plant Guru, and Plant Therapy.

# Cautions

I personally do not feel essential oils should be taken internally. I rely on the plant form for that. A lot of risk resides in the oil purity and processing, but they are also extremely concentrated and would need to be diluted anyway.

I know some brands out there claim purity and internal-use safety. Do your own research, and use your own caution to make the best decision for you.

Some essential oils, like lavender, can be used "neat," or without dilution, safely on the skin. Others, like cinnamon or any of the citrus oils, can cause major irritation. A good rule of thumb is 5% dilution for topical use and 3% dilution for facial use.

Carrier oils are any readily available vegetable oil. I typically use jojoba, coconut, almond, olive, or avocado oil. The carrier oil I choose generally has qualities I want for my face or skin. If not, I pick the cheapest clean option.

## Pet Safety

Below are a few oils to avoid around your pets.

**Dogs:** Avoid heavy citrus, tea tree, and wintergreen oils.

**Cats:** Avoid heavy citrus, peppermint, wintergreen, and eucalyptus oils.

This doesn't mean you can't use them; just avoid them around your pet's water bowls. Don't force the pet in an enclosed area where you're using them in a diffuser. Don't put them directly on their coats.

If using a diffuser around a pet, do your research and only use them in larger areas if the pet has no way to get away from it. Pets will often move away from scents and substances they dislike.

Use caution, research, your best judgment, and pay attention to your pet.

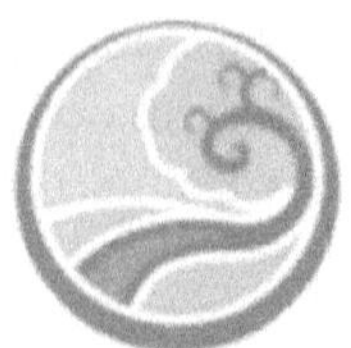

# Roll-Ons

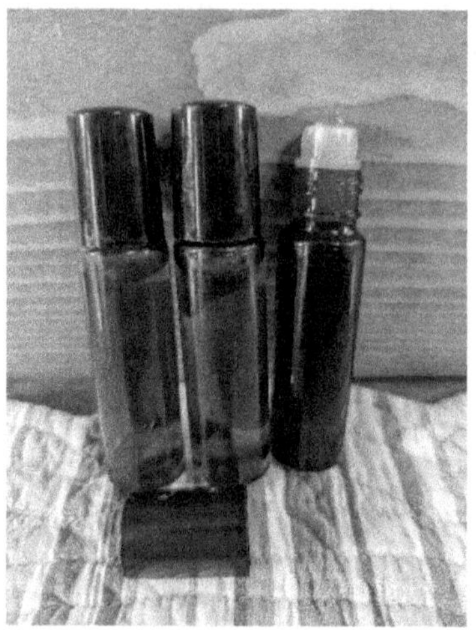

Roller-ball containers are a great way to use essential oils. You premix your oils in the container, top them with some carrier oil to dilute them, toss the container in your purse, or set it around the house for ready-to-go use.

This method can be used for anything from perfumes to hormone balance to relaxation.

Recipes are based on a 10mL roller-ball container. Top it with enough carrier oil to fill the rest of the container, leaving room to pop the roller ball back on.

Most often, I use almond oil as a carrier oil as it's scentless, fairly easy to get, and decently priced.

Remember, these recipes are a place to start. Add or remove oils based on your personal preference, or mix a few things together, with properties that you need, for your own personal blend.

I often find mixes with hormone support helpful for pain relief, as many of us are a little unbalanced.

# Breathe Roll-On

Breathe is my personal blend of essential oils, such as menthol, camphor, and peppermint, for sinus and respiratory pain relief due to colds or allergies. It's also great for sinus headaches.

Apply to temples, base of neck, forehead, chest, and wrist. Breathe deeply.

This is one of my daughter's favorites. She falls asleep directly afterward, as the relief from the sinus headache allows her to relax.

- 30 drops peppermint (contains menthol, offers respiratory relief, pain relief, is invigorating, an expectorant, antispasmodic, decongestant)
- 20 drops camphor (contains menthol, decongestant, offers respiratory relief)
- 10 drops rosemary (helps throat congestion, boosts immune system, reduces fatigue)
- 5 drops eucalyptus (improves oxygen flow)
- 5 drops lemon (improves respiratory function, uplifting, boosts immune system)
- 3 drops tea tree (fights infections)

Other good oils to use:

- Laurel leaf (helps respiratory system, expectorant, decongestant, boosts immune system)
- Cardamom (helps respiratory system)
- Ravintsara (calming, soothes muscular aches and pains, boosts immune system, aids sleep)

# Stress Relief Roll-On

This blend of essential oils is known for its calming and relaxing qualities. It also reduces headaches caused by stress, which is the most common reason I get headaches.

Apply to temples, base of neck, and wrists. Breathe deeply.

- 16 drops lavender (calms, relaxes, releases nervous tension, aids sleep, relieves pain)
- 16 drops vetiver (helps concentration, calming, grounding)
- 8 drops frankincense (elevates mood, boosts immune system, is a sedative)
- 8 drops chamomile (soothing, calming)
- 4 drops rosemary (helps mental focus, boosts immune system, reduces tension and fatigue)
- 4 drops peppermint (invigorating, offers pain relief, gives sense of peace)

Other good oils to use:
- Basil (enhances focus, alertness, reduces anxiety)
- Ginger (fights nausea, soothing, alleviates seasonal affective disorder)
- Spearmint (offers emotional support)

# Balance for Him Roll-On

This blend of essential oils helps men with body aches and emotional balance, especially in regard to hormonal imbalance. It balances hormones and supports healthy emotional and physical well-being.

Remember that even men need progesterone and estrogen, just not in large amounts. These oils help balance the hormones and decrease the pain associated with imbalance and the resulting tension.

Apply to temples, base of neck, chest, and wrists. Breathe deeply.

- 15 drops sandalwood (balances testosterone)
- 10 drops rosemary (reduces cortisol and hormone fluctuation)
- 7 drops peppermint (helps adrenal gland, improves headaches)
- 5 drops clary sage (lowers blood pressure, produces dopamine, estrogen)
- 5 drops thyme (balances progesterone)
- 3 drops geranium (increases adrenal hormone, thyroid hormone, fights depression)
- 5 drops bergamot (increases hormone secretion)
- 5 drops fennel (provides estrogen)
- 5 drops clove (increases testosterone)
- 2 drops cedarwood (lifts mood)

Other good oils to use:
- Frankincense (helps thyroid hormone gland)
- Lavender (helps adrenal hormone gland, stress relief)
- Rose (helps adrenal hormone gland)
- Chamomile (provides stress relief, hormone balance)

# Balance for Her Roll-On

This blend of essential oils helps women with monthly aches, cramps, and emotional balance. It balances hormones and supports a healthy cycle for emotional and physical well-being.

Women need testosterone as well. These oils help balance hormones and decrease the pain associated with imbalance and the resulting tension.

Apply to temples, base of neck, under ears, and wrists. Breathe deeply.

- 15 drops clary sage (normalizes blood pressure, dopamine, provides estrogen)
- 7 drops ylang-ylang (provides estrogen, helps with hot flashes)
- 7 drops rosemary (reduces cortisol and hormone fluctuation)
- 7 drops geranium (helps adrenal hormone, thyroid hormone, fights depression)
- 7 drops thyme (balances progesterone)
- 5 drops peppermint (helps adrenal gland, relieves headaches)
- 5 drops sandalwood (balances testosterone)
- 2 drops vetiver (stress relief, sedative, helps with cramps)

Other good oils to use:
- Frankincense (helps thyroid hormone gland)
- Lavender (helps adrenal hormone gland, relieves stress)
- Rose (helps adrenal hormone gland)
- Chamomile (offers stress relief, balances hormones)

# Pain Relief Roll-On

This blend of essential oils is known to help with nerve pain and improve circulation. This is good for people with arthritis, nerve issues, circulation issues, Parkinson's disease, and restless leg syndrome when caused by nerve damage.

Apply to the affected area, rolling in a circular motion.

- 26 drops birch (relieves pain, boosts circulatory system, reduces swelling)
- 20 drops Helichrysum (relieves nerve pain and stimulates healing)
- 15 drops black pepper (stimulating, increases circulation, removes uric acid, decreases the effect of "cold" pain)
- 15 drops ginger (relieves pain from rheumatoid arthritis and osteoarthritis)
- 13 drops clove (analgesic, anti-inflammatory, pain relief)
- 8 drops peppermint (cooling, joint pain)
- 10 drops orange (anti-inflammation, antiarthritic)
- 6 drops frankincense (helps stiffness)
- 6 drops myrrh (promotes healing, analgesic)
- 5 drops cinnamon (improves motor function)
- 1 full dropperful (approx. 40 drops) arnica (reduces swelling, bruising)
- 2 full droppersful (approx. 80 drops) borage seed oil

# Immunity Roll-On

This immune system-supporting blend of essential oils uses citrus, clove, and cinnamon. It's also perfectly scented to wear in the fall and winter for added protection from the cold-and-flu season.

Hmm, there's probably a reason our ancestors used these scents and spices during those seasons! I can't think about fall without thinking of apple pie or about Christmas without a pomander.

Apply liberally to the chest and bottom of feet after a warm Epsom bath to help fight off illness.

Apply to temples, base of neck, chest, wrists, and bottom of feet. Breathe deeply.

- 20 drops cinnamon (improves metabolic function, immune system)
- 10 drops orange (boosts immune system, contains antioxidants, reduces oxidative stress)
- 10 drops clove (antioxidant, boosts immune system)
- 10 drops myrrh (kills bacteria and stimulates immune system by increasing white blood cells)
- 5 drops eucalyptus (antiseptic, anti-inflammatory, boosts antibodies)
- 5 drops lemon (detoxifying, antiseptic, disinfectant, antidepressant, stimulates white blood vessels to fight disease, circulation)

Other good oils to use:
- Chamomile (reduces stress)
- Bergamot (helps the central nervous system, boosts energy)

- Sandalwood (antiseptic, antiviral)
- Tea tree (disinfectant, boosts immune system, reduces stress)
- Thyme (antioxidant)
- Vetiver (grounding, promotes nerve health)
- Rosemary (detoxifying, anesthetic)
- Clove (antioxidant, soothing)
- Lavender (reduces stress, contains free radicals)

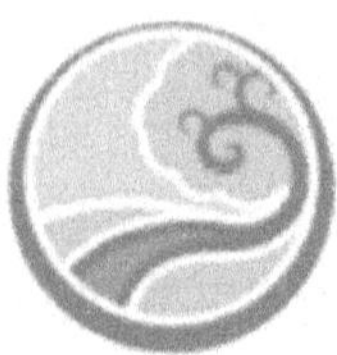

# Diffuser Oils

I really love using diffusers to get essential oils into a room. They are a great way to easily improve the overall health, increase your energy, and improve your sleep. Diffusers also add a little moisture to the air. When airways are moist and healthy, you are less susceptible to microbes invading your body.

However, noticing the growing pile of EOs sitting on my side table, I decided to premix mine (like the Roll-ons) in a dropper bottle. I still have a few bottles sitting next to my diffuser, but they're all blends I know and love, ready to use.

You can find small dropper bottles online, like an eye dropper, and fill them with your own mix of essential oils. Don't forget to label them and keep them next to your diffuser. You should be able to find a pack of them for under $10.

Alternatively, use an upcycled essential-oil bottle. Fill and use as normal.

I use a small dropper bottle, 5mL or 10mL, as these mixes are pure essential oils and larger bottles would be more expensive to make. I use 10mL bottles as they are easier to find, then only partially fill them.

Directions

- Fill diffuser to the max line according to the manufacturer's instructions. Add 5-10 drops essential-oil blend.

*Use the recipes as suggestions. Play around with the scents, and use what you like.

*Note: From Nature With Love: Home and Cleaning Solutions* booklet includes recipes to use as air fresheners, clearing negative energy, calming, grounding, and mood-lifting blends.

## Breathe

Reducing inflammation and congestion in clogged airways helps you breathe more easily and reduces sinus-pain headaches. This mix helps if you are prone to allergies, have breathing disorders, or are just fighting off a cold.

- 60 drops peppermint (menthol, offers respiratory relief, invigorating, offers pain relief, expectorant, antispasmodic, decongestant)
- 30 drops camphor (menthol, decongestant, offers respiratory relief)
- 30 drops rosemary (helps throat congestion, boosts immune system, reduces fatigue)
- 10 drops eucalyptus (improves oxygen flow)
- 10 drops lemon (helps respiratory function, uplifting, boosts immune system)
- 10 drops tea tree (fights infections)

# Immunity

Ward off illness at work or at home by boosting your immune system. Many essential oils are powerfully antimicrobial, and when introduced in vapor form, the organic compounds come into direct contact with airborne pathogens before they can invade your body.

- 50 drops cinnamon (improves metabolic function, boosts immune system)
- 30 drops orange (boosts immune system, provides antioxidants, reduces oxidative stress)
- 30 drops clove (antioxidant, boosts immune system)
- 30 drops myrrh (kills bacteria and stimulates immune system by increasing white blood cells)
- 10 drops eucalyptus (antiseptic, anti-inflammatory, provides antibodies)
- 10 drops lemon (detoxifying, antiseptic, disinfectant, antidepressant, stimulates white blood cells to fight disease, increases circulation)

Other good oils to use:
- Tea tree, sage, rosemary, grapefruit, lemon, thyme

# Stress Relief

Good for tension headaches and stress relief, this is the same recipe mix as the roll-on but used in a diffuser to fully immerse yourself in the relaxation.

Try one at work, at home, during afterwork relaxation, or next to the bed for a better night's sleep.

- 30 drops lavender (calms, relaxes, releases nervous tension, helps sleep, relieves pain)
- 30 drops vetiver (aids concentration, calming, grounding)
- 15 drops frankincense (elevates mood, boosts immune system, sedative)
- 15 drops chamomile (soothing, calming)
- 8 drops rosemary (increases mental focus, boosts immune system, reduces tension and fatigue)
- 8 drops peppermint (invigorates, relieves pain, offers a sense of peace)

Other good oils to use:
- Basil (improves focus, alertness, reduces anxiety)
- Ginger (fights nausea, soothes, combats seasonal affective disorder)
- Spearmint (offers emotional support)

# Sleep

This recipe is in the *For the Home* booklet as a sleep spray, but I also wanted to include it here in diffuser form. It helps achieve a good night's sleep.

- 70 drops lavender (relaxation, reduces tension)
- 30 drops chamomile (sedative, soothing, calming)
- 10 drops vetiver (calming, grounding)

*Note:* Swap out the 30 drops of chamomile with cedarwood for a warmer, woodsy scent. My hubby likes it like this.

# Mood Lifter

Create an energized mood, not just for when you're sad or depressed. This mix can inspire high spirits, set a positive atmosphere before stressful events, or get you moving on slow mornings.

- 20 drops lemon (happy, clarifying, stimulating, improves mood)
- 20 drops sandalwood (calms the mind, soothes stress and nervous tension)
- 10 drops litsea (uplifting, reduces fear, anxiety, nervous depression, tension, and blood pressure)
- 10 drop damiana (fights depression, offers mood stabilization)
- 5 drops cedarwood (boosts confidence, reduces stress, controls emotion)
- 5 drops cinnamon (improves cognition, reduces oxidation, protects dopamine production, improves motor function)
- 5 drops coriander (boosts creative inspiration, positivity, motivation)

Other good oils to use:
- Orange, jasmine, rose, pine, vanilla

# Brain Booster

These essential oils are known for their powerful ability to improve focus, give you a pick-me-up, and level your mood.

Try this diffuser next to your desk at work or on a student's desk at home.

- 20 drops peppermint (cooling, reduces stress, improves focus)
- 20 drops eucalyptus (cooling, fights mental fatigue)
- 15 drops vetiver (soothing, grounding)
- 10 drops lemon (helps concentration)
- 10 drops pine (clears the mind of stress, energizes)
- 5 drops sandalwood (clarifies the mind and helps awaken intelligence, aids in meditation)

Other good oils to use:
- Cinnamon, coriander

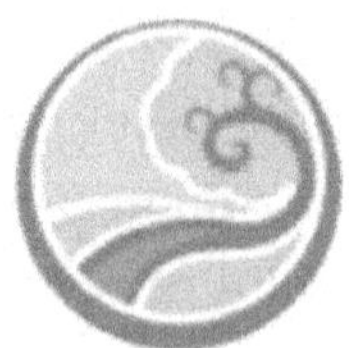

# Poultices

These on-the-spot herbal remedies are the perfect first aid. They're readily available in your backyard or on a hike when you have a cut, scrape, bug bite, or bruise.

Traditionally chewed to a sticky paste, fresh herbs can also be chopped up with a little water and mixed and mashed to the right consistency. You can also plop the fresh herbs right into a clean cloth, dip it in a little hot water, and mash it into a pulp. (If you've hurt yourself, go ahead and work out your anger while you're mashing away.)

Ingredients

- Handful of fresh herbs – below are a few ideas:
    - Yarrow (stops bleeding, bruising)
    - Plantain (soothes bug bites, stings)
    - Comfrey (reduces bruising, muscle strains, and sprains)
    - Calendula (helps heal cuts, scrapes)

Directions – For bug bites, cuts, or scrapes

- The wet, sticky pulp can be applied directly to the wound.
- Either let it dry and fall off naturally or wrap it with a clean bandage.

Directions – For bruises or sprains

- One method is to heat the poultice with a little hot water.

- Put the herbs in a clean cloth or sock and tie it shut.
- Set in a bowl and cover it with a small amount of very hot water.
- Mash the herbs through the cloth into a pulp.

  - Place on the bruise or strain and hold until cool.
  - Rewarm by putting it back in the bowl and pouring more hot water over it. You can also alternate between two packs to make it easier.
  - Continue for 20-30 minutes.

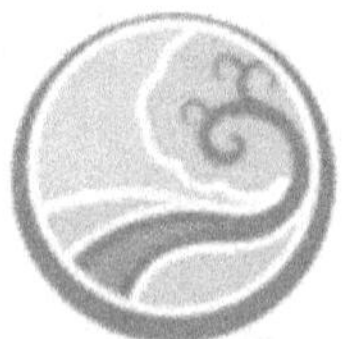

# Seed Cycling for Women

Seed cycling is eating seeds at different stages of your menses to support hormonal balance. Depending on the phase you're in, you eat different seeds for their vitamins, oils, and nutrients.

I'm a big believer in this, and do it regularly. That's not to say you have to seed cycle to be balanced, but it sure does help. I used to only use hemp seeds the week before menstruation to help with breakthrough bleeding but have converted to following the full cycle throughout the month.

Of course, I'm human, so there are times of the year when I slack from it, but I tend to always get back around to it because I believe it helps my emotions and symptoms.

Seed cycling can lessen unpleasant symptoms, balance your periods (more or less if having issues), combat acne, fatigue, sleep issues, infertility, etc.

Add seeds to smoothies, hot cereal, yogurt; sprinkle them on pudding, salads, baked veggies; or bake them into breads or muffins. You can also just pop them into your mouth and chew them up.

Eat 1 Tbl fresh seeds daily, chewing well. Pick your favorite or mix them up.

Some of these seeds spoil quickly. I keep a small container in my kitchen, and the rest goes in the freezer for refills.

Everyone's cycle is different. Ovulation typically occurs at the midpoint of your cycle. Below is a typical 28-day cycle, with ovulation occurring on day 14. Ovulation typically lasts 12-24 hours.

Boost Estrogen – Menstrual and Follicular Phases
Day 1-13 or until ovulation:
- 1 Tbl flax seeds, pumpkin seeds, or raw hemp seeds

*Option*: Grind flax seeds to ensure full breakdown of the seed. This does cause oxidation, reducing its shelf life. Consider refrigeration to lengthen the shelf life of ground flax seeds.

Boost Progesterone – Ovulation and Luteal Phases
Day 14-28 or until menses:
- 1 Tbl sunflower seeds or sesame seeds

*Bonus:*
Days 1-5 (Menstrual)
- Eat warming, anti-inflammatory foods. Ex: Turmeric, ginger, garlic, and salmon (fish oils). Drink red raspberry leaf tea or any other herbs to support your cycle.

Days 6-13 (Follicular)
- Eat foods high in iron, vitamins, fiber, and estrogen. Ex: Leafy greens, seafood, lentils, fermented foods, and nettle. Drink nettle and alfalfa tea.

Days 14-15 (Ovulation)
- Eat detoxifying foods and foods high in estrogen and fiber. Ex: Vegetables, tomatoes, berries, maca, and dandelion roots. Drink dandelion and burdock root tea.

Days 16-28* (Luteal)

- Eat complex carbs to restore your strength and system. This is when your system is resting in between phases. Ex: sweet potatoes, lentils, citrus, dark chocolate (yay!), and root vegetables. Drink chamomile tea.

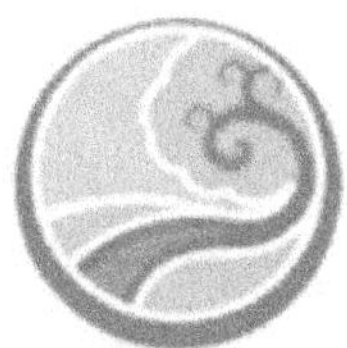

# Cooking with Herbs

Consider adding some herbs directly to your food as nutritional medicines. Sprinkle some nettle or alfalfa into a salad for a vitamin punch, or use red raspberry leaf in a morning smoothie. Herbs are great to add to soups and stews as well.

Get creative and think of additions to boost your family's health or help support organs when healing from a cold or the flu.

Below are a few that I try to add when my family gets sick.

- Black Pepper
- Lemon
- Orange
- Cinnamon
- Thyme
- Marjoram
- Basil
- Rosemary
- Onion & Garlic
- Turmeric
- Ginger

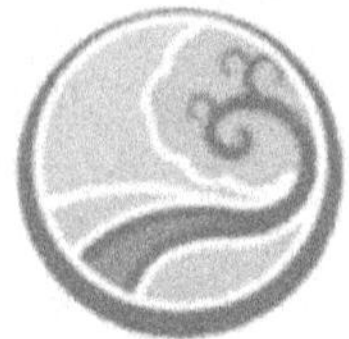

**From the Author:**
Thank you so much for reading this book. After finding my way into natural skincare in an effort to cure adult acne and then longer-term skin health, I realized the benefit of other natural cures. The list is long and the research longer. Luckily, I dream about research projects. I know, my geek is showing.

Fast forward many years, I received my certification in herbalism from The Herbal Academy. I highly recommend them for anyone starting out or wanting to expand their knowledge.

**Author Bio:**
Willa Daniels is a fictional character created by author Jen Flanagan, a certified herbalist living in the Pacific Northwest. If you're interested in hearing more about Willa's adventures with her friends, her newfound magical abilities, and finding love, check out **Saltwater Cures (Orca Cove Series Book One)**.

If you enjoyed this book, the nicest thing you can do is leave me a good review on Amazon, Goodreads, Bookbub, or anywhere you review books.

Connect with me online:
Website: **jenflanaganbooks.com**
Follow Willa on Amazon
Facebook: **@jenflanaganbooks**
Instagram: **@jenflanagan_author**
Bookbub: **@willa_daniels**

Please visit my blog at **jenflanaganbooks.com** for upcoming books, comments, and minor musings.

## What's Next?

I've got several more non-fiction books in the works as part of The Natural Path series. ***An Introduction to Soapmaking*** is out now. ***Home and Cleaning Solutions***, and ***Body and Skincare Solutions*** will be coming soon.

Stay tuned, friends!

<u>Jen Flanagan Fiction Books</u>

**Orca Cove Series:**
Saltwater Cures
Uncharted Waters
Star Crossed (coming 2025)

**Books in the Detective Malone Series:**
Bad Company
Here I Go Again
Under Pressure

<u>Willa Daniels Non-Fiction Books</u>

**Stand-alone books:**
The Art of Living Seasonally

**The Natural Path Series:**
An Introduction to Herbalism
An Introduction to Soapmaking
An Introduction to Sourdough (coming 2025)
Home and Cleaning Solutions (coming 2026)
Body and Skincare Solutions (coming 2026)

www.ingramcontent.com/pod-product-compliance
Lightning Source LLC
Chambersburg PA
CBHW061742050726
47598CB00002B/566